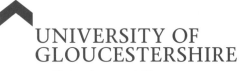

UNIVERSITY OF
GLOUCESTERSHIRE
at Cheltenham and Gloucester

Oxstalls Library
University of Gloucestershire
Oxstalls Campus, Oxstalls Lane, Longlevens,
Gloucester, Gloucestershire GL2 9HW

CARE MANAGEMENT AND COMMUNITY CARE

For Elaine, Tom and Andrew

Care Management and Community Care

Social work discretion and the construction of policy

MARK BALDWIN
University of Bath

Ashgate

Aldershot • Burlington USA • Singapore • Sydney

Published by
Ashgate Publishing Limited
Gower House
Croft Road
Aldershot
Hampshire GU11 3HR
England

Ashgate Publishing Company
131 Main Street
Burlington
Vermont 05401
USA

Ashgate website: http://www.ashgate.com

British Library Cataloguing in Publication Data
Baldwin, Mark
    Care management and community care : social work discretion
    and the construction of policy. - (Studies in cash and
    care)
    1. Public welfare administration - Great Britain 2. Public
    welfare - Great Britain 3. Public welfare administration -
    Great Britain - Evaluation 4. Community health services -
    Great Britain
    I. Title
    361.6'12'0941

Library of Congress Control Number: 00-132613

ISBN 0 7546 1283 X

Printed and bound by Athenaeum Press, Ltd.,
Gateshead, Tyne & Wear.

Contents

Figures

Preface

This book is a record of research exploring the limitations to successful policy implementation. Using Community Care as the illustrative example, it asks what these limitations might be, casting a particular light on the part played by care managers, the front-line policy implementers responsible for "needs assessments" which is a key activity in the implementation of Community Care. There is a tension in care management between the influence of procedures and the degree of discretion necessary for needs assessment to be completed effectively. In what ways, then, are policy intentions affected by the activities of care managers?

Community Care is an illustration of a public policy imposed by central government through a top-down process of implementation in what is argued as a rationalist endeavour to simplify the complexities of community care and reduce it to questions of technique and structure. This attempt to present a unified conceptualisation of community care is backed by managerial procedures referred to in the public management and policy literature as "managerialism". Social work practice theory provides a third example of the rationalist attempt to simplify processes involving complex social interactions.

The limitations to rationalist explanations of community care implementation and the necessity for a different kind of analysis are explored here. There is a parallel with the research methodologies employed for this research. The initial interviews were helpful in revealing the degree to which policy implementation was being thwarted by care managers, but this resistance was mirrored in their rejection of my interpretation of their practice.

The common thread running through the normative approach to policy implementation, management, social work practice and research methodology is an adherence to positivist forms of knowledge. The implementation of Community Care raises questions of epistemology and ontology that undermine these powerful ways of understanding. The claim is that a different epistemology would suggest practices more likely to lead to effective outcomes. An organisational orientation to effectiveness is revealed in the degree to which outcome has become wedded to techniques of scientific rationalism. A service user orientation would define outcome by the degree to which the needs of vulnerable adults were met through reflection upon key relationships. The first of these is an exercise in objectivity which is not well-equipped to take account of the subjective experiences of practitioners exploring needs in relationship with vulnerable adults. The service user orientation suggests an experiential and participative epistemology in which people engage in the process of learning and understanding most successfully when it is collaborative rather than imposed.

Analysis of fieldwork in the second stage involved an experiment using a participatory method of investigation. It gives the reader a glimpse of what might be possible in direct contrast to rationalist approaches. Work with two co-operative inquiry groups has led me to new understandings about the nature of learning for individuals and organisations. The book concludes that an effective learning environment facilitating positive and reflective use of discretion can be created through co-operative inquiry, although any approach would need to include other important participants, notably managers and service users, if it is to maximise its effectiveness in the long term.

Acknowledgements

Many things had to happen to ensure this book appeared in the way that it has. Consequently I would like to thank many people. On the intellectual side, my thanks go to Nick Gould and Peter Reason for their help in providing encouragement and the opportunity for critical reflection throughout the research journey. Linda Challis was there in an earlier phase and was helpful in getting me going. Thanks also to Judi Marshall and Bill Jordan for their constructive challenge to an earlier version.

On the organisational side my thanks go to Elaine Baldwin for all her work in getting the format and layout correct, and also to Clive and Mort for their two penn'orth!

For support and diversion my thanks go to colleagues Nick Gould, Nicki Liles, Jane Batchelor, Sue Barter-Dawe and Karen Boutland, house mates Elaine, Tom and Andrew and music makers Trish, Claire, Will, Andrew, Ben and Mark.

1 General Introduction - Reflecting on the Process

This book is a record of research that has been both theoretical and empirical. It sets out to contemplate the limitations to policy implementation in an environment in which there is room for interpretation of policy through the use of professional discretion by frontline staff within implementing organisations. This has enabled me to make a study of the use of discretion, a subject which has been written about in largely negative terms in the critical literature. The illustrative example is the implementation of Community Care policy during the 1990s, with the empirical work consisting of an analysis of literature, including Local and Central Government documents and direct contact with people involved in the implementation process, primarily at the lower end of Local Government Social Services Department hierarchies (care managers and first line managers). I set out with an interest in knowing how it was that care managers (a key group of professionals in the implementation of Community Care policy) knew what they should do given the bewildering array of knowledge available to them to draw upon in their practice. There is, in what follows, a brief history of the development of Community Care as well as an analysis of the key texts that define the policy intentions of Central and Local Government for the prime tasks of assessment and care management. Empirical work has taken me to meet with care managers and their managers to ask them what informs their practice in carrying out these sophisticated roles, and an interpretation of these meetings is included in detail. Having discovered from this empirical work that not only do care managers find such explanation hard, but also that their practice was in many ways different from the intentions of policy makers, I was then interested in exploring why this should be. This led me on a further journey of exploration providing more information on which I could reflect and increase my understanding.

The book structure can be seen to follow these cycles of action and reflection as my learning and understanding has developed (Figure 1).

Figure 1   **Structure of the Book**

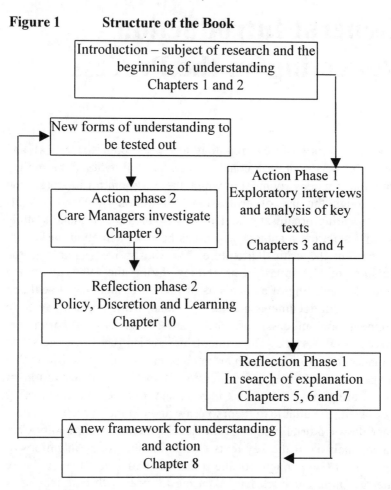

Chapter 1 starts with a general introduction, but also includes a section in which there is a reflection on the personal process of learning involved in this research journey. This justifies the process of action and reflection which is illustrated in figure 1 and provides the structure for the remainder of the book. Chapter 2 offers some contextualisation, taking the reader through some of the problems of policy implementation revealed within policy implementation theory. The chapter is an introduction to the illustrative policy area, and provides the reader with a history of recent developments in Community Care, and the current context in which care managers practice.

Chapter 3 takes the reader into the first period of action. It is an analysis of research interviews carried out with care managers and managers in two Local Authority Social Services Departments. Chapter 4 provides an analysis of some of the key texts which define Community Care. The research interviews demonstrated considerable confusion within the care management field, and the research exploration from that point has been an attempt to explain some of the problems that were encountered. If the interviews provided evidence that policy intentions are undermined by the actions of key implementers such as care managers, it was important to analyse why this should be. The analysis of key texts casts some light on the ambiguities within Community Care policy which add to our understanding of the implementation difficulties. The failure of these documents to provide a single comprehensive version of community care policy which speaks equally to all stakeholders leaves room for interpretation and discretionary behaviour which is likely to undermine intentions when they are based upon policy implementation as a rationalist exercise.

Chapter 5 takes the reader into a reflective phase in which theoretical material is used to address further the problems raised by the interview analyses. It provides a closer look at one key aspect of policy implementation theory, specifically that part that offers an explanation of the role played by front-line implementers. This takes us into the world of Michael Lipsky's Street Level Bureaucrats (Lipsky 1980) and the influence that they can have on policy implementation. Chapter 6 provides an analysis of public service management and the rise of managerialism in public policy during the 1980s and 1990s. The influence of managerialism has been considerable, during this period, and the way in which it has affected policy and practice development has the potential to explain some of the problems facing policy implementation. Chapter 7 puts the spotlight on social work theory. Most care managers are social workers, and it is important to explore what, in theory, might be the forms of knowledge that social workers are drawing upon to inform their practice. Chapter 8 is the last in this reflective phase and analyses 'new paradigm research' (Reason and Rowan 1981) methodology, which has more recently been defined as a 'participatory inquiry paradigm' (Heron and Reason 1997) in contrast to more traditional research within a positivist epistemology. This chapter also provides a link into the final section, reflecting upon knowledge within policy implementation, management, social work and research theory to construct an integrated epistemological framework to help address the main research questions.

Chapter 9 takes the book back into action mode. The coherent epistemological framework developed in the previous chapter is tested out in this one. It is an analysis of two co-operative inquiry research groups which the author was involved in over a six month period with two groups of social workers operating as care managers. These co-operative inquiry groups enabled me to test out the usefulness of experiential participative research methodology and other forms of knowledge to understand the complexities of policy implementation.

Chapter 10 is the final reflective section and provides conclusions in the form of present learning and future action in policy implementation, the use of professional discretion, and organisational structure and management. Some claims are made for the usefulness of participation and reflective practice as starting points for both the study and implementation of policy in a context of organisational learning. It is argued that participation and reflection are more useful than the rationalist and positivist approaches analysed earlier in the book.

How practice differs from policy intentions is of great interest to a number of people, and there is information within the book that covers that ground. It is not the prime focus, however, which is more on *whether* care managers have an influence on policy outcomes and *why* it happens in the ways discovered, and *if* it has to be like this. There is also a case made for a more effective methodology for investigating these questions. I have used a range of theoretical perspectives to help explain why this happens and to explore some of the implications for the future, both in terms of further research and future implementation practice. It is important to ask why it is of interest to know whether care managers can skew policy implementation through their discretionary behaviour. There is a view expressed that there is some inevitability that policy will be determined more through frontline workers' practice rather than from the top down. If that is the case then presumably frontline workers - care managers in our case - would want such influence to be positive and developmental, adding to the quality of service and advocating the values, knowledge and skills that they believe to be important and effective. Evidence of the unbridled and unreflective use of discretion suggests that, for a number of reasons, care managers do not have a controlling hand on the way in which their practice determines policy outcomes. More deliberate and considered use of discretion might, along with the introduction of other practices, actually make service delivery more effective from a number of perspectives. That is why it is important to explore whether care managers skew policy implementation, why and how this happens.

The whole book, though, is rooted firmly in the empirical work - and most notably the two periods of fieldwork. The first involved a close look at the practice of care managers and the second, engagement in a process of practice development with two groups of practitioners. Both these forms of fieldwork - the snapshot and the process - tell us much about the whether, the how and the why, as well us being a useful evaluation of research methodology as it shifted from a traditional qualitative approach to a participative action orientation.

The book starts with the big questions. "What are the limitations to successful policy implementation?" and, more specifically, "are policy intentions undermined by frontline or "street level" implementers?" There is also a third question assuming that the answer to the second is "yes". The additional question is - "what better explanation is there for understanding the actions of street level implementers which might provide a model for more successful implementation?"

The problem that continually raises its head is that of rationalism. Whilst in no way wishing to undermine our status as rational beings who have to make sense of our lives in structured ways, I have struggled, in this journey of exploration, to understand why it is that rationalist forms of social action, based on positivist epistemology, hold such powerful sway in all the key areas of exploration - policy implementation, organisational and managerial structure, professional practice and research methodology. We need to explore if policy can be implemented through rationalist means, whether informed by policy implementation theory at the macro level, scientific managerialism at the mid point or traditional social work theory at the micro level. The problem is not so much that scientific rationalism is used to explain these areas of interest, but that its construction of a particular form of reality through the powerful deployment of discursive practices (Parker 1992) or persuasive rhetoric (Majone 1989; Soyland 1994), is largely unquestioned outside of academic reflexivity.

Positivism is the philosophical approach to epistemology that accepts a unified conceptualisation of reality describing what we all experience and can agree upon. Scientific rationality is the form of social action that involves uncovering, revealing or responding to the objective reality construed by positivist epistemology. Rationalism then creates practices and institutions which are based upon this objective reality. By ignoring the 'important problems' that positivism glosses over (Berger and Luckmann 1966; p. 210), rationalist social action is unable to take account of the ways in which any form of social action constructs, or legitimates, the realities which are more helpfully viewed as 'symbolic universes' (Berger and Luckmann 1966; p. 210). There is much support for this critique of positivism and scientific rationalist social action, notably within the field of social work theory and practice both implicitly and specifically, from a range of perspectives or viewpoints including reflective practice (Schon 1983, 1987; Laragy 1996; Fook 1996), feminism in social research (Gregg 1994), existentialism (Thompson 1995), post-modernism (Howe 1996) and critical reflexive approaches to the evaluation of practice (Shaw 1996).

It is my intention to investigate some of the problems created by these rationalist institutions because of my observation that policy is implemented by people through processes of interrelationship, within organisational structures. People, with their multitudinous and messy ways of making sense of everyday life, create these relationships and organisational structures in a far more fluid and relativist way than rationalism, as defined above, allows. The constructivist version of reality is built upon an uncertain and contingent epistemology. It requires an exploratory and flexible approach to learning. It has revealed to me, in my process of learning, the problems that the clarity and certainty of rationalism create. Assuming the reality is there to be found, it constricts the range of possibilities, failing to acknowledge that what is actually happening is a continual and fluid construction of social reality. Rationalism is not searching for truth but constructing it. The essentialist assumption, however, means that the search continues in unacknowledged, unreflexive and assumptive fashion. Rationalism is, therefore, linear in its process of making sense, and blinkered in its field of vision.

In this book I investigate rationalist approaches to policy implementation, organisational process, management, professional practice and research methodology, and deconstruct the powerful realities, or 'symbolic universes' that they have created within the focus of attention - Community Care implementation. I pose claims to new paradigms in the forms of knowledge that help us make sense of these areas. I am tackling, therefore, some of the 'important problems' ignored by positivist rationality in this area of investigation. The main problem is the use of discretion and the way that its use in policy implementation constructs a different version of policy to that intended by policy creators. Discretion by care managers can then be viewed as the social construction of one form of social reality for Community Care. Discretion is an activity which has been demonised as professionals out of control, requiring increasingly technocratic responses to regain authority by policy implementers higher up the implementation hierarchy. There is no reason, I wish to argue, why discretion should not be seen as a more constructive opportunity to implement policy such as Community Care, as a co-operative and participatory activity.

I started out on this enterprise as a solo traveller. In the latter stages, I realised that it was important to work alongside others making sense of the puzzling area of focus, to collaborate with a group of people who wrestle with the ambiguities and confusions of 'the swampy lowlands' (Schon 1987) of community care on a day-to-day basis. Ultimately we all have to make our own sense of what lies before us, and to act on that knowledge. My emerging belief that we create our real world in relationship with others has led me to realise that empirical work is most usefully carried out co-operatively. There is, in the latter stages of this book, a description and analysis of two co-operative inquiry research groups (Heron 1996) that I engaged in with care managers in a different local authority from the first fieldwork event. Both the process and outcomes of these inquiries have proved very fruitful in extending understanding of the two major focuses for this book - the philosophical question of how we (best) construct useable knowledge, and the political question of how policy intentions can be realised through implementation practices.

I end with the writing of this book, as I started, in individual mode, making my own sense of the journey. One of the things I have discovered along the way is that unless we can apportion and combine our differing views, and work participatively towards a shared understanding, we lose two major opportunities. The first is the opportunity to acknowledge and respect other people and their *difference*. The second is to learn from difference, using knowledge created, in a continuous developmental practice. 'Research is for us' say Reason and Marshall (1987; p.112). 'It is a co-operative endeavour which enables a community of people to make sense of and act effectively in their world' (Reason and Marshall 1987; p. 112). These simple statements differentiate research as a participative process from the positivist approach of objective detachment of the knower from the known. Interestingly enough it also echoes much of the rhetoric of community care in the requirement on local authorities to establish the

collective needs of the communities they serve. This rhetoric also speaks
of services being determined by local authorities in collaboration with, and
taking account of the expressed needs of, ordinary people in the
community. It is this kind of congruence between different forms of
knowledge that it is important for me to pursue. This is my purpose as a
learner and that is one of the reasons why I have followed the process
which has been described. Reason and Marshall (1987) point out that
research needs to speak to three audiences - for them, for us and for me.
For my own integrity I have learnt that this is the way I need to do it, for
the sake of authenticity I have learnt that it needs to be that co-operative
endeavour - creating useable knowledge together. If others wish to use the
results of research, how much better that they should understand that it was
founded on an 'authentic and complementary research process' (Reason
and Marshall 1987; p.113).

Reflexive and Reflective Research - Justification of Process

An explanation of the process of the research as revealed in this book is
important at this stage. A book should not just be a piece of academic
output but should reveal the author as a learner. This is not a post-hoc
rationalisation, but reflection on a process of inquiry and learning. I am
persuaded of the need to be both reflective - 'showing ourselves to
ourselves' (Steier 1991; p. 5) and reflexive - 'being conscious of ourselves
as we see ourselves' (Steier 1991; p. 5). There are powerful arguments in
professional practice (Boud et al 1985; Schon 1984; Schon 1987; Gould
and Taylor 1996) that practitioners such as social workers should be
reflective both in and on their practice. Researchers are no different in this
case and we will look at that later in this section.

To be reflexive 'implies that the orientations of researchers will be
shaped by their socio-historical locations' (Hammersley and Atkinson
1995). To be 'insulated' (Hammersley and Atkinson 1995) or disclocated
from the object of one's research, or to pretend that we can be objective in
that sense is to construct an inauthenticity which is likely to undermine any
validity claims. My reflexiveness has been continuous throughout the
process of the research. It is helpful to take a moment to record this
because of the degree to which my understanding of my part in the
construction of research findings has affected and shaped the process of the
research. I have been reflexive about my position not only as a researcher
and academic but also as a teacher of social workers and as an ex-

practitioner and manager of social work. All these factors influence my perspective on the subject in question.

My 'socio-historical location' as a researcher is affected by the weight given to research within an academic environment. This plus the marginalisation of social work research within a School of Social Science, and Social Science within a broader technical University provides a pressure on the social work researcher which is palpable. How is it possible to prove oneself as a *real* researcher in this context? This, plus my awareness of the traditions of research in the social work arena were hard to ignore. The safety of the positivist paradigm in social research, and the tradition of qualitative research methodology heavily influenced my entrance into the first fieldwork component of this research. This becomes part of the explanation if not the justification for qualitative research interviews which are described and analysed in Chapter Three. Reflexiveness is a permanent revolution, however, and, along with the reflection which I will describe below, induced the realisation that there were different ways of understanding social research. Modernist and Post-modernist analysis of social work practice and theory (Parton 1994; Howe 1994) plus the literature around participative action research methodology (Reason et al 1981) enabled me to understand a different way of seeing myself as a social work academic in my 'socio-historical location'.

As an ex-practitioner and manager, and as a teacher of future social workers I was aware of a further reflexive arena. In carrying out my research, both through a review of the literature and in fieldwork with practitioners and managers, I have tried to maintain my awareness of these aspects of self-identity. The desire to make a case for social work as a practice for care management within community care, was both supported by the literature and undermined by the explanations I heard in interviews. I was acutely aware of the wealth of knowledge, skills and values within traditional and contemporary social work theory that could be used to both guide and justify practice in care management, whilst at the same time greatly frustrated by the inability of the care managers I interviewed in the first period of fieldwork to articulate this knowledge base. I drew heavily upon my experience of being a practitioner and manager in similar social services departments at times of great change, recognising and empathising with the way interviewees revealed their grasp held firmly on the known in the face of the new. I heard the expressions of powerlessness in the face of the organisational machinery, and I felt my own rising empathy and irritation in almost equal measures!

To have assumed my objectivity in this process would have been to be blind to the bias. We have to 'understand the cultural forms through which "truths" are accomplished' (Silverman 1993), in order to disentangle the knower from the known.   Silverman postulates four forms of 'sensitivity' to qualitative data including 'contextual' in which phenomena mean different things in different circumstances and where different meaning creates particular contexts.   In this situation, he argues, 'authenticity is more important than reliability' (Silverman 1993; p10). Being aware, therefore, of this context of differential meaning over a period of time means that research is about 'social phenomena as *procedural* affairs' (Silverman 1993; p.29).   My interviews with practitioners and managers were then 'displays of perspectives and moral forms' (Silverman 1993; p.107) revealing not scientific truths but versions of reality. As a reflexive researcher I need to ask "why *this* reality in this context?" As an ex-practitioner myself and as a teacher and researcher I approach this with some knowledge of a historical perspective in which we can see the evolution of ideas and forms of knowledge which inform certain organisational practices and practitioner responses. A researcher with a different biography would almost certainly have made a different sense of the same material. Validity, then in this sense is more about recognising and reflecting upon the reasons for such differences, and not about attempting to establish some unifying truth.

My reflexiveness is about both the way in which knowledge and truth is constructed and also about how persuasive that knowledge can be. As a beginning researcher swayed by my position in a fairly hostile research environment, needing to prove my credentials, I opted for a traditional qualitative research methodology. On reflection, I realised that there were other ways of constructing useable knowledge and most notably in participation with co-subjects in research, rather than doing research on and objectifying subjects as happened with the initial interviews.

The term reflectiveness defines the process by which this happens. As with cyclical approaches to learning (Kolb 1984) reflectiveness is 'a form of response of the learner to experience' (Boud et al 1985; p. 18). Boud and his colleagues add that 'it is only when we bring our ideas to our consciousness that we can evaluate them and begin to make choices about what we will and will not do' (Boud et al; p.19) The key words with reflection then are that it is integral to *learning* , that it is a *conscious process of evaluation*, and that it is related to *experience* or *doing*. We will return to the concept of reflectiveness, which became a considerable area of learning in its own right, later in the whole process, in Chapter Seven. For now it is worth noting the usefulness of Boud's model for the process of reflection as, in hindsight, it helps explain the direction that my research journey took me. Reflection is about 'returning to experience', 'attending to feelings' and 're-evaluating experience' (Boud et al 1985; p.26). The part of the process to do with returning to experience in research evaluation terms may seem a truism. The point, for reflective practice rather than more scientific approaches is to ensure that it is the *experience* which is reflected upon and not an objectified version of it. It will be seen that those taking part in the initial research interviews participated in the findings to virtually no degree whatsoever. This lack of response to the (beautifully crafted) research document which I passed to all involved had a fairly devastating effect on me at the time. I needed to be aware of this emotional response and use it as a dynamic for learning and moving forward rather than for closure. The result was a particular approach to the third aspect of reflection - the re-evaluation of experience. What transpired was the search for a different and more participative methodology for the second period of fieldwork. This process of reflection explains why I opted for the changed methodology described in Chapter Eight.

Paradigms for inquiry activity (Guba 1990) can be characterised by response to three questions. Firstly there is the ontological question - 'what is the nature of the "knowable"?' (Guba 1990; p.18), secondly the epistemological question of the 'nature of the relationship between the knower and the known' (Guba 1990: p.18), and thirdly the methodological question of how the inquiry should go about finding knowledge. I have found myself to be a naturally reflective and reflexive researcher who, having acknowledged this, has sought to develop relevant skills. Such reflection has taken me to the heart of questions about the knower and the known, and enabled me to be more sophisticated, as time has passed, about the 'regulative ideals' (Schurandt 1990; p.269) which determine chosen methodology. Schurandt cautions against the 'primacy of method' (Schurandt 1990; p. 272) and suggests that 'fidelity to subject matter' and 'complementarity' (shared knowing) (Schurandt 1990; p. 272) are these ideals. It is not possible, I would contend, to know what fidelity or complementarity are in practice without adopting the reflexive and reflective approach argued for in this section. It is important that this is born in mind in reading the remainder of the text.

What I have attempted in this book, therefore, is a record of a development of understanding owned by myself but (in latter stages) carried out in participation with others.   It is to that extent a record of 'colluding with others to create new knowledge' (Carlen 1996) as a colleague helpfully put it.   It has been interesting for me to note the way in which my developing understanding has resulted in a congruence of approach, in which the nature of inquiry, the nature of policy implementation and the nature of social work (reflective practice) are all informed by the same epistemology and the same participative philosophy. This is reflected in the structure of the book which takes the reader through cycles of action and reflection (Figure 1).   It also explains the use of a range of methods, most notably between the fieldwork approaches of the first and second contacts with care managers.   Co-operative Inquiry followed semi-structured interviews after reflection upon the learning that resulted from the latter.

2 Policy Implementation and Community Care

Introduction

I have already described this book as a theoretical and empirical study of policy implementation. I am concerned to explore different forms of explanation of what has been termed 'implementation deficit' (Pressman and Wildavsky 1973). What are the limitations to policy implementation? Why is it that policy implementation is never *perfect*? In particular I wish to examine the practitioner influence on policy implementation, and to ask other questions – *are policy intentions undermined by the activities of implementers? How do those involved in implementation - especially social work practitioners in the illustrative example of community care - construct a body of knowledge that is of use to them in carrying out the implementation process? What other factors influence the way they behave?* As a social work academic, responsible for providing an education for future social work practitioners I make no apology for this micro approach, although I recognise that the broader picture is also important. This chapter starts with a broad analysis of policy implementation theory before looking at the illustrative policy example of Community Care.

If we contend that it is right that policy implementation can be skewed by practitioners, what evidence is there that supports the contention? This has been the principle concern of the 'bottom-up' policy implementation theorists who provide explanations for policy outcomes which are of interest to someone who wishes to explore the influence of practitioners. Just how persuasive are other policy implementation theorists, in particular rationalists, in their explanation and their models for practice in policy implementation? If it is true that practitioners are of influence and that rationalist explanations are insufficiently persuasive then what might be a better way of a) explaining what happens in policy implementation and b) developing a more effective method of implementation? This book will provide views on these subjects and justification for them.

Policy Implementation Theory

Policy implementation theory is a much contested area. The literature (Hill 1993; Hill, M 1997; Hogwood and Gunn 1984; Hill and Bramley 1986; Ham and Hill 1993; Lindblom and Woodhouse 1993) provides some interesting tensions which are helpful in exploring and understanding what is happening within the illustrative policy arena - community care. The principal tension is between the claims of rationalist analysts and others who argue against the certainties of a positivist approach to implementation theory. Majone (1989) argues against the scientific model of policy analysis that requires 'formal proofs' (Majone 1989; p.2) by introducing other factors that are neglected in rationalist theory, and need to be considered in policy analysis and, therefore, implementation. He claims that 'inference' and 'articulation of values' are equally valid, producing what he terms 'multiple policy evaluation' which recognises the 'legitimacy of different perspectives' (Majone 1989; p.9). He refers to policy analysis that claims to be value free as 'decisionism'. This scientific approach fails to address the process through which differences of perspective are articulated. This is a political and participative process, and the ways in which some voices are allowed to be articulated and others not regulates the degree to which power is wielded in the political process. The process of decision-making is described by Majone as 'mutual learning' (Majone 1989; p.41). This connection between policy making and learning, and its description as a *process,* is an important concept that will be reiterated and expanded upon in this book. It is a notion that is well supported by the literature on organisational learning (Argyris and Schon 1996), in which it is argued that an organisation's identity is largely accounted for by the construction of 'theory-in-use' by members of the organisation working in relationship together. As Green and Zinke have noted, Majone's view of policy implementation as a political process results in the construction of 'rhetorical ways of knowing' (Green and Zinke 1993; p. 317). Failure to appreciate that perspective and value are articulated in a process of rhetoric or persuasion in policy implementation, means that scientific rationalist theory is unable to reveal the complete picture when it makes the positivist claim that human action can be understood objectively and outside of the person, without taking into account their interests, their perspective or their values.

Another tension in policy theory is revealed in the differences between 'Top Down' and 'Bottom Up' approaches to implementation. It is this area of tension which provides the somewhat spurious battle between the virtual reality of rationalism (Hogwood and Gunn 1984) and the more descriptive approach of those whose analysis focuses on the activities of implementers at the bottom end of the implementation hierarchy. Top Down theory, which has been described as a rationalist approach (Lindblom and Woodhouse 1993) is built on an assumption that, given the correct forms of implementation process - guidance, procedures, organisation, training and (especially in the past twenty years) management - policy implementation will proceed as intended by implementers at the top of organisations or Government. This is a prescriptive and normative approach designed to assist those interested in implementation to understand the best way to proceed.

Bottom up analyses are more descriptive of how things are, although those who advocate such an approach would also claim that it provides the same opportunities for advice to implementers. This perspective on the policy process offers us two forms of guidance to understanding and action, despite all the constraints on policy implementation. Firstly we need to think of implementation as decision making within 'successive limited comparisons' (Lindblom 1988; p188) and therefore incremental in nature, and secondly to study the behaviour of key implementers. The latter argument takes us into the realm of Street Level Bureaucrats (Lipsky 1980), and is explored in greater depth in Chapter Five. It is particularly the issues of discretion and accountability that are explored in Lipsky's conceptual arena, and provides us with a contrast between different forms of legitimacy within policy implementation. Lipsky also helps us to understand the way in which policy is constructed by implementers, particularly at the street level in organisations, although there is an argument that this occurs throughout organisations that are more or less successful at generating an environment of organisational learning (Argyris and Schon 1996). Lindblom's incrementalism also provides a critique of rationalist theory, noting that there is seldom such a thing as new policy. Community care is an example of a policy that builds on a considerable history of policy initiatives that have been tried and tested and to which different constituents, or stakeholders, will attach varying value. It is the failure of rationalist or 'synoptic' (Lindblom 1988) approaches to address this concept of value that also reduces their effectiveness in providing anything more than an *ideal-type* for policy implementation theory. This partial explanation for important areas such as organisational behaviour and most notably the actions of 'street level' (Lipsky 1980) implementers, limits their usefulness.

The problem with Lindblom's incrementalism is that it provides an excuse for inertia, is fundamentally conservative (Smith and May 1980) and 'favours the strong' over the weak (Ham and Hill 1993). Attempts to produce some sort of hybrid between rationalist and incremental approaches, such as Etzioni's 'mixed scanning' (Smith and May 1980), in which a broad sweep of policy is followed by incrementalism at the decision-making stage does not really get beyond this favouring of the status quo. Lindblom argues that incrementalism is best understood as a process of 'partisan mutual adjustment' (Lindblom 1988; p. 252) in which differing perspectives are introduced to the policy process in much the same way that Majone argues (Majone 1989). The problem with Lindblom's analysis is his failure to address power relationships in policy implementation. He does not offer any convincing argument to explain the process by which some perspectives are permitted in the decision-making process and others are marginalised (Bachrach and Baratz 1970; Lukes 1974). These arguments will be returned to at a later stage, but it is important to contrast the difference between Lindblom's rejection of rationalist implementation assumptions and his preference for 'successive limited comparisons' (Lindblom 1988; p. 188).

A third tension is that between prescription and discretion. At the macro level, matters will always intervene to influence and even frustrate the intentions of Government in prescribing a particular policy formulation (Hill 1993c). These interventions will be matters such as local autonomy which legislators have to take into consideration when drafting legislation. The failure by central Government to resolve some of the political dilemmas posed by a policy or the use of ambiguities to create localised forms of information are also likely to frustrate intentions. Community care is a good example of this. A look at the policy guidance for care management (Baldwin 1998) reveals the degree to which different agendas are being addressed which result in a lack of clarity with regard to political, procedural and practice intentions.

These are heinous sins for implementation practice according to the rational theorists (Hogwood and Gunn 1984). Clarity of goals, simplicity of organisational structure and control over implementing actors are the key variables that policy implementers at the top will need to ensure are under control if 'implementation deficit' is to be avoided. The problem for the rationalist certainty which underpins this top down approach is that even the most prescriptive standards for practice have to be interpreted. A form of 'Chinese Whispers' in which intentions are passed from Department of Health to Social Services Inspectorate to social services departments through management hierarchies to practitioners provides several layers of interpretation resulting almost inevitably in a shift away from original intentions. In the pursuit of more efficient techniques of implementation, rationalists will argue that there must be reliability of prediction which can be assured through having the key variables listed above in place. Reliability requires rules and regulations, and it is notable within our illustrative example of community care, that such regulations have proliferated in the years since Griffiths was commissioned to produce his Report (Griffiths 1988). Rules and regulations, however, create rigidity, and rigidity denies flexibility. In order for procedures to deliver the services necessary to create the reality of community care for those for whom it is intended - service users - flexibility is essential. Effective services, according to Government policy, have to respond to individual need (D of H 1989) and an individually tailored service requires flexibility. Flexibility of response by welfare bureaucracies inevitably means allowing some degree of discretion to staff, particularly those (care managers) who are primarily responsible for assessment and care planning. The way that the rationalist argument for reliability through the implementation of increasingly rigid rules unravels in the face of the complexity of need and the requirements of a discretion-based flexibility, fundamentally undermines rationalist, top down prescription for policy implementation. This is not to dismiss the importance of rules and procedures for policy implementation. As will be seen from the empirical work within this book, procedures are clearly important in guiding the use of discretionary activity and ensuring that practice proceeds down a broadly similar pathway and, therefore provides equity and equality of treatment. The problem is of the primacy of procedure over practice within a model of implementation that assumes the correct technocratic approach will produce the required outcome consistently.

A further tension in implementation is between regulatory coercion and pluralism. Where there is ambiguity in policy definition as there is in community care (Baldwin 1998), the degree of political will for implementation becomes very important. An example of this within community care is the concept of service user empowerment. There are many different versions of this concept, often argued within the broader concept of citizenship (Ramcharan, Roberts, Grant, and Borland 1997; Beresford and Croft 1993; Adams 1996). We have seen the development of a clear distinction between a concept of citizenship based on new right consumerism within a market economy and the maximisation of citizens' rights through self-determination. How coercive ministers and the Department of Health wish to be in regulating the behaviour of social services departments to ensure market structures are implemented is mirrored by how coercive local authorities want or are able to be (through managerial systems) in regulating whether key implementers such as care managers behave as entrepreneurs or purchasers in the new welfare market.

One further tension which has developed in more recent years with the burgeoning service user movement, exists between the arguments for democratic accountability (i.e. the actions of elected politicians) and the weight given to the *voice* of service users. Politicians may feel they have some justification in arguing that it is they who have a responsibility to determine policy derived from their electoral mandate. This notion is increasingly challenged by the concept of participatory democracy in which other stakeholders - users, carers and professional service providers - have been encouraged to demand a say. Indeed this concept is written into the community care legislation through the requirement on local authorities to consult with their communities and voluntary organisations when they put together their Community Care Plans. This is another example of the ways in which the top down and bottom up arguments are played out.

Rehearsing these arguments between different versions of implementation theory and practice reveals a number of useful contentions. Firstly there is a body of thought - rationalism - that influences policy implementation practice by its claim to prescribe implementation procedures which will ensure that change can proceed as closely as possible to the way intended. The flaws that have been noted in these arguments should in no way detract from the extent to which this rationalist approach is revealed within such discursive practices as care management systems, priority matrices and eligibility criteria. Evidence for these practices can be found in Government guidance, reflected in local authorities' policy guidance (see Chapter Four for a full analysis of this guidance). There is a second body of thought which argues specifically against this rationalist or 'synoptic' (Lindblom 1988; p. 242) approach, preferring instead explanation and practice that considers the incremental nature of implementation (Lindblom 1988) and the influence of implementers such as practitioners on the development of policy. The seminal work in this latter area is Lipsky's "Street Level Bureaucracies" (1980), and his book will be used as a major source of theory to analyse empirical work in Chapter Five.

There is another, more recent, body of knowledge, that argues the usefulness of post-modernism as a critique of rationalist explanations of policy implementation. The deconstruction of the metaphors of control by Dobuzinskis (1992), is one example of this. His postmodernist analysis of the policy process suggest that these metaphors of control too often 'convey the image of policy 'makers' in control of their environment' (Dobuzinskis 1992, p.374). This image, he argues, is becoming less credible as a way of making sense of 'problem situations where there is insufficient knowledge about cause and effect relations, and where societal actors are capable of acting in unpredictable ways' (Dobuzinskis 1992, p.374). Using the same conceptual framework, Schram (1993) argues that 'linguistic practices help construct and maintain personal identity' (Schram 1993, p.249). This presents us with a very different approach to welfare recipients - service users - in contrast to the objectivist labelling process that occurs within rationalist implementation theory. This analytical perspective becomes more persuasive in the face of 'the growing ranks of political actors who distrust technocratic discourse' (Dobuzinskis 1992, p.374).

Whilst offering a critique of top down implementation because of its adherence to rationalist ideas of certainty, and its failure to accept the central part taken by actors in constructing policy on a day to day basis, we must return briefly to the point made earlier that this is a somewhat spurious battle. The tensions between competing explanations for policy implementation are a helpful rhetorical device whilst trying to make sense of complex processes, but it is important to note that there is an issue of responsibility and accountability here. Clearly policy makers at the top of organisations, especially within government, have a responsibility to construct and present policy for acceptance by all interested parties. Such policy initiation should be top down, assuming that there has been an acceptable degree of consultation and participation in its construction. This is what is expected. Initiators of policy need to have engaged in a degree of consultation that persuades implementers and recipients of policy initiatives, because, if they do not, they will encounter resistance, either in the form of activities described by Lipsky (1980) as those of street level bureaucrats or in the form of protests by potential service users that we have seen in recent years by disabled people campaigning against the failures of policy makers to address their needs. As Pottage and Evans have noted 'there is an urgent need to build on and negotiate policies based on the everyday meanings and understandings that are created by the interactions of workers and users.' (Pottage and Evans 1994: p. 16) They later argue that 'events have their meaning in the way they are experienced', a phenomenological perspective which is at odds with the normative hierarchical culture that assumes the positivist certainties that 'events and decisions will be the same wherever they are located: hence the tendency to define practice from the top down.' (Pottage and Evans 1994: p. 60) So the problem is less to do with the position from which policy is initiated, it is more to with the positivist assumptions, the hierarchical organisational processes and the authoritarian imposition of policy. Policy implementation would, therefore, more usefully be seen as a process of negotiation, both at its formulation stage and during its implementation. I contrast this concept of policy negotiation through participation with the top down rationalist version of implementation which is more aptly defined as imposition through the mobilisation of powerful political forces.

All the above arguments help reveal the contested nature of policy analysis, exposing the weaknesses of rationalism as a valid explanation, and presenting some alternative approaches that favour a version of policy analysis that views it as part of a socially constructed human reality (Berger and Luckman 1966). It is this notion of the social construction of human reality together with the concept of agency (Long and Long 1992; Giddens 1976) which helps explain the part that important actors such as care managers can and do play in the construction of community care. These arguments lay the foundation for the following sections of the book, in which empirical research is firstly described and then used to test out the extent of practitioner influence on policy development. The rest of the book provides further opportunity for debate about the relative merits of these different perspectives as we make sense of the contested policy arena of Community Care.

Community Care and Care Management - the Context for Exploration

This substantial area of government policy provides the illustrative example of the broader research arena that is proposed at the beginning. Although the phrase community care has been around for some time, there is little doubt that the primary context in which people think of these words is that of health and welfare services for adult service users. This is what is meant by community care in this book. It is argued, therefore, as the policy and practice that flows from the White Paper 'Caring for People: Community Care into the 1990s and Beyond' (D of H 1989) followed by the implementation of the National Health Service and Community Care Act of 1990. It is important to note, however, that this legislation appears within a historical and political context and both the act and the guidance which has emanated from it are evidence of a process of action and understanding which is continuous and connected. Community Care as we now understand it, was not built on a green field site (Challis 1996).

For the purposes of this work we need go back no further than the end of the war, and in no greater depth than to note that the process we now refer to as community care or care in the community developed from a desire to shift the balance of care from large Victorian institutions to smaller units of residential care and the provision of community and domiciliary care services as alternatives for people who are able to remain living in their own homes as opposed to institutional care.

This occurred with the shift in care for older people from some of the former workhouse accommodation into residential care as defined under Part Three of the 1948 National Assistance Act. For those who lived in large psychiatric hospitals, the Mental Health Act of 1959 provided the authority to shift the emphasis of health and welfare services in a similar direction. Care for those who had learning difficulties was also shifted from hospital to residential care, largely as a result of some notable scandals about the quality of care in hospital settings (Means and Smith 1994).

Debate about the motivation for these shifts in the location of care from absolute or 'total institutions' (Goffman 1961) to institutions within the community has been considerable (Means and Smith 1994; Lewis and Glennerster 1996; Malin 1994). This would seem to suggest that change probably occurred as a result of a complex convergence of influences rather than from one particular effect such as, for instance, cuts in Government spending, or a welfare inspired shift from institutional to more homely and community based care for vulnerable people. The sources above also argue that this change was more of policy than of practice. The resources that were intended to replace the asylum (at its most gentle and non-pejorative, a word meaning sanctuary) by services in the community, never really materialised. This is still the case today, particularly in relation to mental health, where a move from psychiatric hospital into 'the community' calls up images of frying pans and fires.

This raises the issue of definitions. The argument, at its simplest, is between the concept of care in the community - the most appropriate form of care for each individual, with all services, whether day care, domiciliary or residential striving to play a fuller part in the 'community' - and the concept of community care - in which day and domiciliary services are seen as separate and 'better than' residential care, which is, by this definition, *not* in the community.

There is a clear tension in the historical development of community care between the normative liberal values of closing outmoded and oppressive institutions such as "mental handicap" hospitals, with the influence of fiscal crisis within the welfare state which demanded the same resulting policy initiatives and practice. This tension helps to explain many of the contradictions and ambiguities in community care policy, and the way in which the same policy - closure of long-term institutions - can speak to constituents with very different sets of values. It is important to note that, as with many other aspects of community care, there are differences of opinion, of emphasis, of value and ideology, which reveal community care as an area of contested meaning. Research into this area needs to be able to deal with these shifting sands of meaning and this is justified both in the next section of this chapter and through the analysis of government documents in chapter four.

The Audit Commission (1992a) takes community care to mean non-residential care. There are people involved in the delivery of residential care services, and striving to make them relevant and appropriate for at least some people for whom it has been a 'Positive Choice' (Wagner 1988), who find this definition, this 'reality', undermining of their enterprise. This is exactly the point of this analysis. How do these different perspectives work together? How can they be *managed*?

The changes in policy and the half-hearted practice that followed, were largely instituted in the 1960s and 1970s. They have had an effect on the position as we experience it now. The changes which occurred in the 1980s and increasingly in this decade, however, have been far more radical and fundamental. These more recent changes can be traced (Means and Smith 1994; Lewis and Glennerster 1996) to the political transformation that occurred following the election victories of the Conservative Party between 1979 and 1992. These governments signalled a shift in ideology from the post-war consensus on health and welfare service delivery to a new ideology dominated by neo-liberal or new right views of economic and social relations.

The divergence in government policy from a dominant reliance on state provision of services, to a position where local authorities in particular (in this context) are under pressure to purchase services from the 'independent' sector has become irresistible. The obligation to do this has come from both legislation and central government guidance (for example the insistence that LASSDs spend at least 85% of their funds transferred from Social Security as a result of NHS and Community Care Act implementation in April 1993 within the 'independent' sector). Services are now increasingly drawn from a 'mixed economy of care' (D of H 1989) with Social Services Departments less and less able to continue the provision of their own services.

The common theme of neo-liberal political and economic ideology may be clear in these developments, but, as with the earlier developments noted above, the actual influences were more complex, being pragmatic and ideological in equal measure. The deregulation of social security funding for residential care in the early 1980s, largely argued from the ideological grounds that disabled people should be able to choose private care if they so wished, led to an astronomical and uncontrolled rise in the use of this form of care, which cost the tax payer very dearly indeed.

Expenditure in this field rose from £10 million in 1979 to £459 million in 1986, and it was still rising into the 1990s (Means and Smith 1994).

At the same time as this development, the government were showing every intention of wishing to reduce local authority influence in areas such as social services. This development in private residential care can be seen from this point of view as well, but it had the effect of severe criticism by the Audit Commission (1986) and the House of Commons Select Committee (Social Services Committee 1985) for failure to control public expenditure.

The acknowledgement by government that something had to be done about this state of affairs culminated in the appointment of Sir Roy Griffiths, former head of Sainsburys, to look at the whole arena of what was now classified as 'community care'. The appointment of someone who was defined as a successful manager within a private sector enterprise was symbolic of government ideology at work. There was a firm belief within government that imposition of the rigours of the market and the expertise of those who had triumphed within it were the only ways forward in providing welfare services that people wanted (the political imperative) and which were cost effective (the economic imperative).

The Report produced by Griffiths (1988) was a mixed bag for the government. It fully endorsed the ideology of the market place, insisting that the introduction of quasi-markets (LeGrand and Bartlett 1993) was the best way forward for social services as, it was claimed, it was proving for health. The control of welfare services, however, was to be located within the local authority, with social services departments taking the lead. That this recommendation did not accord with the government's desire to curb the power of local authorities explains the delay in the response to Griffiths' Report. That they finally accepted it largely intact, is an indication of the political pragmatism that the Conservative government demonstrated in the past and somewhat undermines the 'pure ideology' rhetoric that was sometimes used against them.

Social welfare services were eventually defined within the limitations of the White Paper, Caring for People, which was published in 1989, and have since become enshrined in the legislation of the NHS and Community Care Act of 1990, and by the guidance that followed (SSI 1991 a and b). The content of these and other key texts in the development of community care is looked at in much greater detail in Chapter Four but, for the purpose of introduction, it is important to spell out the key objectives of government policy as revealed in the White Paper in particular. These were sixfold. The government wished to 'promote the development of domiciliary day and respite services to enable people to live in their own homes' (D of H 1989; page 5) where this was possible. Secondly 'practical help for carers' was to be made a priority. Thirdly 'assessment of need and good case management' was to be 'the cornerstone of high quality care'. Fourthly, it was intended that 'the development of a flourishing independent sector' should be promoted. Fifthly, systems to 'clarify responsibilities' should be established so that LASSDs could be more easily held to account. The final intention was to 'secure better value for taxpayers' money'.

Much has been written since this White Paper in the way of policy (D of H 1990) and practice guidance (SSI 1991a and b). There has also been a weight of literature from local authorities, clarifying their interpretation of government intentions either to local constituents in the form of statutory Community Care Plans, or practice guidance documents. There has, in addition, been much written in the way of critique of government policy from the academic and professional lobby (Means and Smith 1994; Lewis and Glennerster 1996; Malin 1994), but the White Paper remains the best document if we wish to establish a normative view of Community Care in practice. The care management model, in essence, is there. Some of the structures that have developed since, within Local Authority Social Services Departments (LASSD), to support care management and the assessment of need are also firmly rooted within the text of the White Paper.

Community Care in the Context of this Book

Anyone with a fleeting interest in community care will know that, even with the strength of the White Paper's definitions, it is an area of contested meaning. Community care will mean different things to different people, depending, in large part, on their relationship to the organisation of service delivery. Given that community care is a phrase used to define a huge swathe of government policy it would clearly be useful to establish a more sophisticated idea of what the government means by it. This might then explain what they intend to happen, as well as give us a yardstick by which to evaluate what has actually emerged. The pursuit of meaning is an important part of social work practice. It is a fundamental tenet of good social work practice that social workers should ensure that they have understood what service users mean in describing their perspective on their condition. There are times when social workers have to impose their views on unwilling service users, but, more often than not, they are trying to understand and respect other people's sense of meaning. What follows is not exclusively about the social work practice of understanding meaning, although, in one sense, that is exactly what assessment practice is all about. It does, however, acknowledge that varying meanings exist. This argument is expanded upon in detail in Chapter Four.

In order to contain this book within the enormity of a subject like community care, the area that will be focussed upon is the assessment task within care management.   Following the publication of the White Paper 'Caring for People' (D of H 1989) and the enactment of the NHS and Community Care Act 1990, Local Authority Social Services Departments have been required to introduce new structures for organising the delivery of services to adults in the care sector. This has resulted in the universal introduction of systems of 'care management' in social services departments.   In order to assist the process of introducing care management into departments, the government, through the Social Services Inspectorate, produced manuals of guidance for both practitioners and managers.   The Department of Health and the Social Services Inspectorate also commissioned the National Institute of Social Work to produce a practice guide. These three documents have been influential in social services departments, most of which have produced their own documents of guidance.

Prior to carrying out the first phase of fieldwork for this research, therefore, I had an idea of what the government's intentions were in relation to care management. The White Paper and the Policy Guidance (D of H 1990) that went with it provide the major policy thrust of government intentions, introducing the key concepts of the community care 'revolution'.   The fundamental changes were concerned with introducing an internal 'quasi-market' (LeGrand and Bartlett 1993) into the adult services arena of social welfare, following a similar introduction into the National Health Service. This internal market was believed by the government, informed by a market economy agenda, to provide the best way of introducing choice of high quality services targeted on those who are in greatest need.

In order to ensure that there is no contamination of the market ideal, those responsible for the purchase of services on service users' behalf should be separated from those within Social Services Departments who are responsible for providing services. Hence, as in the NHS, purchasers of services (those carrying out assessments and putting together care packages) should be in a separate part of the organisation from the providers. Indeed, there is a strong incentive for social services departments to relinquish their traditional role as service providers and to develop a mixed economy of care through the encouragement of the independent sector (private and voluntary).

Care management, along with assessment, has been presented, by the Department of Health as the key form of practice for introducing these changes into the provision of adult services. The definitive versions of care management can be found in the guidance documentation (SSI 1991a and 1991b). The Practitioners' Guide and Managers' Guide have been heavily influential on social services departments in preparing their own guidance documents for care managers. That there are problems of consistency, especially in the area of role definition in these versions of care management requires greater analysis, and this can be found in Chapter Four. Having read the government documentation as well as having studied 28 social services department care management guidance documents, I was keen to establish the extent to which the knowledge embodied in the documents was being used by practitioners to inform their practice. This was the fundamental purpose of the fieldwork described in the next chapter.

The Department of Health through the Social Services Inspectorate has produced a definition of care management (SSI 1991a) which is analysed in considerable detail in Chapter Four. For now, a description of this process is required as it is important as an influential part of the context for community care. Having read 28 of them, it is clear that this document has provided the model for most of the care management guideline documents produced for their care managers by local authority Social Services Departments. Very few of the guidelines I have studied deviate from the SSI document in any way at all. They habitually define care management as a cyclical process, following the model in Fig. 2. Thus providing information in accessible forms to potential service users, and a system for determining the level of assessment to be offered following referral are the pre-requisites to the cyclical process suggested. A number of local authorities have decided not to follow the option of having levels of assessment, choosing instead to offer a blanket assessment to all who are referred. There is evidence, however (Baldwin 1995) that there is confusion amongst care managers as to whether their authority is sanctioning "levels" of assessment or not. The third stage, of assessing need, is the key stage according to the guidance. The summary of practice guidance urges care managers to look at 'strengths and aspirations' (SSI 1991a: p.11) as well as needs, calling on care managers to bring together contributions from other agencies and specialists as appropriate. Needs are to be assessed 'in the context of local policies and priorities' (SSI 1991a: p.11) which are part of the information to be published in stage one. The care planning stage number four requires care managers to present appropriate resources available from both statutory and independent sectors to enable the potential service user to make a choice of services which would then constitute a "care plan". In stage five the care plan is implemented through negotiation by the care manager with appropriate agencies, including their own. It is also the stage at which financial negotiations are instituted so that responsibility for payment for the package of care can be confirmed. The final two stages, which feed back into the assessment process, involve monitoring the care plan and then regularly reviewing its effectiveness, in the context of service user's and carer's unfolding needs over time. The monitoring would be continuous and is likely to involve service providers keeping the care manager informed of progress. Reviews will occur at specified intervals and would involve care manager, service providers as well as users and carers. These stages would have a general quality assurance function in the 'continuing quest for improvement' (SSI 1991a: p. 11) in the merits of the services provided as parts of the package of care. This structure is the normative approach to care management in community care. As suggested above, there will be further analysis of this model, both in theory, in chapter five, but also in practice in chapter four.

Figure 2   **The Care Management Cycle**

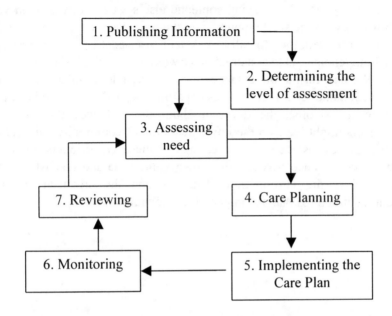

The importance of role clarity within a task as complex as assessment has not prevented it from becoming a contested arena in its own right. What the research that informs this book has sought to do is seek out the variety of meanings and the forms of knowledge that inform the practice of assessment within care management. We can then draw tentative conclusions about the range and degree of influence that different types of knowledge exert on practice, and their affect on the implementation of policy. If there is no congruence between the knowledge and values that inform the policy implemented through local authority departments and that which informs the practice of frontline practitioners, then it is likely that there will be a gap between intention and practice leading to 'implementation deficit'.

This is a central line of argument within contemporary social welfare. The tension between professional, political, and managerial approaches to service delivery can perhaps be better understood within this context. The voice of users and potential users of welfare services can also then start to find a space within which it can be heard in its many guises. If assessment, as many Learning Difficulties (Souza 1997 in Ramcharan et al) and Mental Health service users are now telling us, means the oppressive experience of having someone else's views foisted upon you, your own view of the world denied, and the way you wish to run your life disrupted or altered, then to call assessment 'user-centred', 'empowering', or 'enabling choice', is to construct an Orwellian style doublespeak.

We now turn to the evidence provided by talking to care managers in two local authority social services departments. This evidence is helpful in trying to establish the question about the influence that frontline practitioners might have on the implementation of community care policy. It also provides insight into the feelings of these practitioners about the degree of congruence between their own value base and that which they believe drives the introduction of policy and the organisational and procedural structures that accompany implementation.

3   Care Management and the Subversion of Policy

Introduction and Aims of the Research Interviews

This chapter[1] analyses interviews that took place in 1994 with 30 managers and care managers involved in the management and practice tasks that are essential to the continuing implementation of community care policy. There is, in what follows, a statement of the aims of the interviews, a description of the participants and the methodology, followed by analysis of the contents of the interview transcripts. Further reflection on these interviews follows from Chapter Five, when a range of theoretical perspectives are used to try and make sense of the methodological, epistemological and practice problems encountered in the analysis of this first piece of fieldwork.

Before describing and analysing this period of fieldwork it is important to locate it in the process of research that constructs the whole of the book. The analysis which now follows was drawn from the fieldwork carried out within the two agencies whose staff were interviewed by me. I am seeking to maintain the flavour of that report in much of the description and analysis within this chapter, because it is important that I try and describe the way that I was thinking *at the time*.

The preconceptions that I started out with, and which I needed to be aware of, are documented within this chapter. There is some post hoc rationalisation in some parts of the chapter, but I have kept that at the level of contextualisation and only in the places where I believe it is helpful as explanation. My surprise at the outcome of the interviews - my interpretation of what I heard care managers saying to me - was genuine and constitutes an important part of the process of my learning for the whole book. It also had a direct influence on the direction that the research subsequently took and which is documented within the book. In my

---

[1] A similar version of this chapter appears as Baldwin, M (1995) *The Meaning of Care Management*, Social Work Monographs; Norwich, University of East Anglia

analysis of the interviews I experienced a range of reactions to the evidence which comes in the form of anomalies, surprises, patterns familiar to me as an experienced practitioner and manager, depressing confirmation of other research material that documents examples of poor practice (e.g. Ellis 1993; Audit Commission 1992a) as well as validation of dynamic and developmental practice within care management.   These things were all evident in what I learnt from listening to managers and care managers in the two local authorities.   I need to document my learning without too much post hoc rationalisation, so that the reader can see why it was that I moved on to explore these anomalies and puzzles in the way that I did.

There was a substantial gap between what I might have expected to have heard care managers were doing when carrying out assessments having read the policy literature, and what they actually described to me. That needs explaining, but I am, as will be seen, not content in only explaining.   It is also important to me to explore how things might be different, and, most particularly, how practice which is so fundamental to implementing community care policy might be more effective.

The fieldwork interviews did, however, provide an early opportunity to address the research questions.   Entering into discussions with care managers and managers working in the adult care services of two local authority social services departments provided an opportunity to look at the part being played by key implementers, many of them working at the "street level", in the implementation of community care policy.   It was early days following the enactment in April 1993 of those parts of the National Health Service and Community Care Act which were to have the greatest effect in the organisation, management and practice of needs assessment.   One year on from this enactment I was hoping to make some judgements from these interviews of the degree to which policy intentions were being realised as intended or frustrated by other factors.   The state of knowledge about implementation at that particular time suggested that some of the key features - needs-led assessments, service development and service user involvement, were being frustrated (Ellis 1993; Audit Commission 1992b).   Research suggested that implementation was being blocked as a result of the actions of practitioners (Ellis 1993) and poor systems of management (Audit Commission 1992b).   My research questions were interested in addressing the blocks to policy implementation generally, but with a particular focus on the activities of street level implementers.

One of the potential limitations to policy implementation according to the rationalists, is policy coherence. Even prior to this fieldwork, and prior to the more detailed analysis of documents dealt with in the next chapter, it was clear to me that there are different kinds of knowledge revealed in the government publications that define community care policy [2], and, therefore, that care management and assessment were concepts with contested meaning. There seemed to be a managerial agenda involved in care management which was concerned with the importance of cost effectiveness, resource control and value for money (Bamford 1989; Pollitt 1990). I also identified a professional agenda that was more concerned with issues like empowerment, the formation of relationship to aid the exploration of problems, and the active use of theoretical perspectives to inform practice (Smale et al 1993). Increasingly there seemed to be a service user orientated approach (Taylor et al 1992; Beresford and Croft 1993) within the influences revealed in the literature. This agenda introduces concepts such as user involvement both in individual assessment and in the broader perspective of resource development. Finally, I also noted a political agenda (The White Paper (D of H 1989) is the best example of this) that borrowed from these other three to some degree, using the language of managerialist and professional approaches, as well as that of user involvement, to produce a hybrid agenda, designed to sell changes to political constituents who would include managers and professionals as well as local politicians, the general public as well as potential users of services.

Caught up in the midst of these competing agendas are the care managers who are required to carry out assessments and put together packages of care in negotiation with service users. What were they making of these competing influences on their practice? Which, of the different types of knowledge, are they most likely to draw upon to inform what they

---

[2] The publications chosen for this purpose are listed below. Justification for the choice is made in the following chapter.

Audit Commission (1992) *The Community Revolution: Personal Social Services and Community Care,* London, HMSO

Department of Health (1989) *Caring for People: Community Care in the Next Decade and Beyond,* London, HMSO

Social Services Inspectorate (1991) *Care Management and Assessment: Managers' Guide,* London, HMSO

Social Services Inspectorate (1991) *Care Management and Assessment: Practitioners' Guide,* London, HMSO

Smale G, Tuson G, with Biehal N, and Marsh P, (1993) *Empowerment, Assessment, Care Management and the Skilled Worker,* London, HMSO

do when carrying out a sophisticated task such as assessment? Were there other, as yet unidentified, forms of knowledge that they were using? The forms of knowledge that care managers were drawing upon would provide evidence of the degree to which they were implementing policy as intended, although, as has already been stated and will be established in even greater detail in chapter four, policy intentions are not altogether clear in the most significant literature.

Research Methodology

Choice of Authorities

Between April and September of 1994 interviews were carried out with staff in two local authority social services departments. Originally it had been intended to carry out interviews in three local authority social services departments which conformed to notional points on a continuum of adherence to central government intentions with regard to the introduction of an internal market in social welfare. I was looking for an authority that had pursued the intentions explicitly at one end of the continuum, another that had resisted the intentions and complied with the minimum of statutory requirements at the other, with another authority at the midpoint on the continuum. Unfortunately the authority chosen for the midpoint pulled out of co-operation at a late stage, and after letters of introduction had been sent out. It was too late to renegotiate another similar authority and I chose to continue with only two, which did, at least, afford a direct contrast and comparison.

One of these authorities was a London borough (identified hereafter as Borough) and the other a shire county (to be known as Shire). Shire had pursued the government agenda from an early stage, making an organisational divide between purchase and provision earlier than most other Social Services Departments. This meant that the staff in the authority should have already gained considerable experience of the kind of organisation and practice changes that care managers in other authorities, like Borough, had only been used to for one year. Borough, on the other hand, were recommended to me as an agency who were following government guidance only so far as statutory requirements insisted. A comparative study between these two agencies was chosen on the grounds that there was sufficient differentiation between the two departments to provide useful comparison and establish a degree of validity in the findings.

After the interviews, I studied the care management guidelines from Shire in order to establish what level of congruence there might be between the intentions of that document and practice in the department. Borough did not have a similar guidance document, but relied on the Social Services Inspectorate guidance (SSI 1991a; 1991b) on care management as the reference point for practice. My principle focus was on the actions of care managers in their role in the *assessment* of potential service users' needs. Inevitably, however, I needed to have some knowledge of the whole care management cycle within which assessment sits, as it is perceived of as a whole within the literature (SSI 1991b) rather than a fragmented part. This cycle was described in Chapter Two (p. 65ff) and is further explored in Chapter Four.

The Participants

Interviews were carried out with care managers and first line managers in both social services departments. In addition two middle managers in Shire, and one senior manager in Borough were interviewed to obtain the view of staff with budgetary control and strategic responsibility within the agencies. In Borough, interviews were carried out with 8 staff doing assessments within adult services. Three of these, as well as carrying out assessments themselves, also had first line managerial responsibility for other staff carrying out assessments. Of these 8, 3 were qualified social workers, one an occupational therapist, and the others had no formal qualification but with training and experience appropriate to the task. I also interviewed three other first line managers in Borough, who had responsibility for the management of teams of workers. Two of these were qualified social workers and one an occupational therapist. Finally, in Borough, I also interviewed a senior manager in one 'area' who had budgetary accountability, responsibility for managing first line managers, and strategic responsibility within the area and the whole borough.

In Shire I interviewed 9 care managers carrying out assessments. Two of these were child care workers, the rest worked in disability teams. All were qualified social workers except for one who was an occupational therapist and another who had the diploma in domiciliary care management. I also interviewed 6 first line managers in Shire who were responsible for budgets and managing care managers. One of these managed a child care team, the rest were managers of disability teams. All were qualified, one as an occupational therapist, and the rest as social workers. The two middle managers in Shire that I interviewed were both qualified occupational therapists. They had staff management, budgetary and local strategic planning responsibilities. The gender of participants was mixed in both Authorities, and in each grouping of workers. Ethnicity was varied in Borough, but all the interviewees in Shire were white. I noted the ethnicity of interviewees as I felt the possibility of black perspectives on care management might reveal a different approach to the task from their white colleagues.

The Method

The interview schedule was semi-structured, comprising a list of questions that everyone was asked, but with the option of follow up questions, in order to seek clarification where necessary. I maintained a checklist of potential responses that I could prompt interviewees with, should they have problems in answering questions. I was very aware of the problems, in using interview schedules, of misunderstanding. Foddy (1993) from a symbolic interactionist perspective casts doubt upon the usefulness of responses because the 'relationships between what respondents say they do and what they actually do is not always very strong' (Foddy 1993; p. 1). It is very important then, to ensure that the questions are understood in the way intended by the researcher and the answers, conversely, are understood as intended by the respondent. There were important issues of meaning and intention that I was aware of, and determined to avoid the pitfalls of misunderstanding. Other writers on qualitative research methodology (Silverman 1993; Lindlof 1995) urge the importance of interpretation and the need for piloting before and checking out during interviews to avoid the worst excesses of a 'scientism' (Silverman 1993 p.2) and 'abstracted empiricism' (Silverman 1993; p.27). I concurred with Silverman, and did not believe that bias could be 'techniqued out' of an interview schedule (Silverman 1993; p.29), rather seeking to remain vigilant, questioning and flexible in order to proceed with as few assumptions as possible. Prior to the research interviews in Shire and Borough I piloted the interview schedule in a team from a nearby local authority.

When I started the interviews in Shire and Borough the flexibility I was seeking proved invaluable as it rapidly became apparent that individual workers were fulfilling more or less subtly different roles in different settings, sometimes with the same job title. This was particularly the case in Borough, where decentralisation had created structures within different 'areas' which were very particular to that patch. The fundamental purpose of the interviews, to get at the actual practice of individuals, and compare it with what policy and practice guidance told them they 'ought' to be doing, made the avoidance of assumption a basic value of the research interviews. In a similar vein, it was important that individuals were able to speak freely and in confidence about their work, and the organisational context, again, so that the degree of congruence between the 'ought' and the 'is' could be gauged. Confidentiality and anonymity were 'de rigeur'.

Meaning Revealed

The interviews were all tape-recorded and have been transcribed. The transcripts have been studied in detail, and key themes have been extracted through content analysis. In what follows all quotations in double inverted commas (" ") are direct quotations from participants. In order to avoid being guided purely by my 'hypothesis', that there are limitations to policy implementation as a result of the activities of key implementers, I have looked widely for issues that have arisen, and group them under three different headings:

- *Role of the Care Manager*
- *Use of Procedures and Resource Management*
- *Implementation of the Principles of Community Care*

It should be noted that I had no access to the outcomes of individual's practice in this research, only what they said about what they did. I have used care managers' own words where that is illustrative, but the interpretation is mine.

1. Role of the Care Manager

Under this section we can look at the influences on their practice that interviewees listed. How do care managers see their role? What are the knowledge, skills and values that they believe inform what they do? What might the difference be between professional backgrounds, or between those with a qualification and those without?

Influences on Practice

I started by asking a general question 'what influences your practice?'. A substantial range of responses was revealed, and I felt that these 'volunteered' responses were at least as significant as those made to prompts about specific influences on practice.   The most frequently mentioned pre-checklist responses were factors like "instinct", "gut feelings", "the personalities involved", and "experience".   Agency procedures - filling in the forms - was also a frequent response, but training, either in-service or professional was less often stated as an influence on practice, prior to respondents being given a specific opportunity to comment on this.   Even when training and theory were offered as prompts, many respondents found the question difficult. Only very few quoted specific theoretical models that they use to inform their practice or by which they evaluate what they have done. One or two of these answers were very impressive, the rest seemed somewhat embarrassed by their inability to dredge up theories they had learnt on training programmes, often some years before. Some practitioners were able to articulate models of practice even though they could not put a name to them.

As far as comparisons between Shire and Borough, qualified and unqualified, social worker and occupational therapist are concerned, there was not a significant difference when the initial question was put. Qualified workers, when given the opportunity to speak of theory were generally better able to do so.   There were some notable exceptions, mainly where unqualified staff had made excellent use of prior learning, or in-service training to inform their practice, and were able to cite particular theories or models that they used to inform their actions.

The question of the relevance of training to the task of care management is an interesting one.   There were some responses that indicated a feeling that social work training was not relevant to care management, but most did not make a judgement on this. A senior manager in Borough felt that the current teaching on diploma in social work courses was inadequate for the role, but still the best available.

Most assessment practice seemed highly problem focused. This was particularly the case with occupational therapists. Again, there was very little difference between Shire and Borough in this analysis. It is important to add that the unqualified workers practice in this regard was at least as well informed as the qualified social workers. Some unqualified staff spoke most eloquently about the practice skills involved in needs-led and user orientated assessments.

'Resources' were given as an influence on practice in two different ways. Lack of resources influenced practice in general, but so did knowledge of available resources. This left me with some concerns about the degree to which assessment outcomes were being determined by what care managers believed were the resources available to meet any apparent need. We shall return to this point later.

One of the clearest differences between the two authorities concerned the degree to which 'values', 'attitudes', equal opportunities or anti-discrimination were volunteered as influences on practice. In Shire, these were seldom mentioned before the prompt. Even after Shire care managers were prompted with the question about values as a potential influence on their assessment work, many still volunteered little in the way of response that indicated a widespread understanding of a need to be influenced by, for instance, concerns that some service users may be disadvantaged in particular ways. There were some notable exceptions to this from care managers qualified for some time as social workers.

In Borough, on the other hand, there was almost universal volunteering of the need for ethnic sensitivity, taking cultural difference into consideration and other similar practice values. This was primarily the case in relation to 'race' as a potential area of disadvantage. This sensitivity was perhaps not surprising given that in one of the Borough 'areas' the black population was set at 60% by one care manager. Borough care managers were also more likely to think of equality of opportunity in relation to age, gender, disability, sexual orientation and poverty than their counterparts in Shire. I felt that this level of difference was likely to have an effect on practice. Care management guidance documents from government and local authorities urge consideration of such factors so failure to do so would indicate divergence from policy intention, as well as a less effective assessment outcome.

Several qualified social workers in both Shire and Borough seemed uncomfortable about their difficulty in articulating values in relation to assessment practice - "I realise I haven't really thought about values for ages, it's terrible". There were, as before, exceptions to this point, with some impressive articulation of values by some individuals (qualified social workers from both agencies and unqualified care managers from Borough). In addition, some teams had well defined and shared values in relation to their practice, the most impressive example of this being in Shire - "as a team we have a stated document which list our aims and values ... an absolute commitment to equal opportunities ... working towards anti-discriminatory practice ... recognising that we do discriminate". The sort of values that were referred to in these cases are in the form of a set of principles to which social workers - in this case as care managers - are committed and which inform them of how they *should* behave (Banks 1995). The Central Council for Education and Training in Social Work (CCETSW) is the body that validates and provides regulations for professional social work courses. CCETSW's current statement of value requirements (CCETSW 1995) includes such phrases as respect for diversity, building upon strengths, promoting rights to choice, confidentiality and protection, countering discrimination and assisting people in increasing control over and improving the quality of their lives. This area of values is returned to in Chapter Seven when social work theory is looked at in detail.

In conclusion it was apparent that of the many influences on practice in assessment, not all relate either specifically or even incidentally to policy guidelines. There was evidence of unconsidered reliance on intuitive approaches to practice - "a lot of gut feeling, a lot of intuition, you've just jolly well got the vibes". The apparent failure to reflect on the origins of this knowledge, added to some resistance to formal sources of knowledge and values - "I don't think I consciously draw on anything, I just think that I do things"; "I've forgotten all these things (theories and models) they all go out of your mind"; "I'm certainly not comfortable talking in the value thing - we're almost getting into mission statements" - makes congruence between policy and practice less likely.

Assessment - Knowledge Skills and Values

Assessment was focused upon in this research because it is argued as a key area in the care management cycle (Social Services Inspectorate 1991b). We have already looked at some of the influences on practice. There are other issues of practice and role. Care managers almost invariably indicated the need for assessments to be needs-led, and for the individual to be the focus of assessment. There was revealed, however, a very widely held belief that service users are not really interested in participating beyond an assurance that they will receive the service that will meet their needs. This was justified through sentiments such as "I think a lot of service users don't understand". Time constraints on involvement were also revealed - "It really does take time, I mean time and effort to involve people"; "the reality is that you can't sit around and do it with them". This apparent failure of involvement has resulted in care managers adopting a role which shifts away from maintaining the service user at the centre of the assessment exercise. The likely result is an assessment based more on their professional opinion than on an assessment formed through partnership. Using this evidence we can question the extent to which care managers allow their role to be defined by what they believe users want as opposed to what community care policy, procedure and ethos suggests is good practice. User involvement requires the education of service users into greater expectations, as much as it requires the education of staff into new ways of thinking and practice. This was clear evidence of a gap between the intentions of community care policy and the practice of care managers. It is interesting to note that the *values* of service user involvement are contemporary social work values (CCETSW 1995) as well as policy intentions.

Care Management - Procedure versus Practice

My questioning found some debate amongst first line managers in both agencies about two models of care management. Most care managers seemed less interested in defining a new role and more with protecting those parts of their current practice which they hold dear - "I'm actually doing very much the same thing as I always was". The two models were referred to as the "procedural" and the "laissez faire". Also referred to at one point was the "exchange" model from the NISW book which is described in detail in the following chapter (Smale et al 1993) and which takes us close to the good practice intentions of CCETSW requirements. The procedural model was perceived as mechanistic, following agency bureaucratic guidelines, and involved little active reflection on the nature of the relationship between worker and user. The other model is based more on traditional social work as a practice, and involves the forming of relationship and the use of this for exploration and problem solving. In the NISW book there is a similar model of assessment, referred to as the "questioning" model. This model also holds with a basic assumption that it is the care manager's role to make the judgement, based on their professional expertise.

Although care managers did not talk directly about these models, they are a helpful way of differentiating the forms of practice to which care managers appeared to hold allegiance when they described their aims in carrying out assessments during interviews. Some care managers clearly wanted to continue an approach to assessment built on the use of relationship, as they felt they had always done, and resisted the introduction of bureaucratic techniques as a consequence - "I believe these forms are a barrier between a person and an assessor"; "if you present those (forms) to someone, the walls are up straight away". These tended to be care managers who had been qualified as social workers for some time. It is my view that this practice was closer to the questioning model, which involves a more traditional application of professional knowledge, than the exchange model which defines assessment and care management practice within a participative context. There were few care managers from both Shire and Borough who seemed to be using anything resembling the exchange model. Those who did were the same care managers who were clearest about their role, and seemed to be practising nearest to agency requirements in the Shire Guidance document. Other care managers seemed happier with a procedural model, indicating that they would like the assessment instruments to be more prescriptive: "The forms are just blank pieces of paper", complained one respondent.

I found this debate to be evidence of confusion of role in both agencies. It may be that there is room for different kinds of care manager in a department, but the difference in perceived role does have an effect on practice, particularly in relation to user involvement in the assessment process. The perception of role confusion by care managers in both authorities has a detrimental affect on confidence and results in care managers sticking to what they know and feel assured of rather than moving on into a new and uncertain practice about which many have both concerns and suspicion.

Some first line managers suggested that recently qualified workers were more likely to adopt a mechanistic approach to assessment - "what I find with more recently qualified staff and with student social workers is that they are looking at assessments in a much more mechanical, administrative, bureaucratic way". This was a good critique of contemporary diploma in social work teaching, and there was some limited evidence for the assertion. On the other hand, there were also examples of exchange practice from newly qualified staff, and, generally, it was hard to associate the approaches to any one group - social workers, occupational therapists, or unqualified workers. One manager made the interesting point that she believed procedural models were "undermining the traditional instincts" of care managers. She was referring to the use of relationship by social workers. There was also a direct contrast revealed between professional and procedural models of assessment, with the interviewee being clearly in favour of the former - "ability to communicate, relate and set up a relationship will be a factor which is not a very measurable factor". This resulted in resistance to the procedures to demonstrate that favour in practice - "there are some people who will try and get round the procedures because they feel they are working against the best interests of the client". This was actively encouraged by some managers - "so I said to her (an anxious social worker) forget the forms, just remember how you make a relationship with an old person ... it (use of the forms) totally deskills some of the most experienced workers in the team".

In both Shire and Borough there was a strong defence of procedure from two care managers who were impressively clear about their role (the Shire care manager was social work qualified, the Borough one was unqualified). Both of them, interestingly, whilst advocating a user focused and needs-led assessment practice, insisted that bureaucratic procedures introduced an element of equity into practice that had been very patchy in the past - "you've got the same set of forms and everyone gets the same ... and you look at the needs"; "I personally feel about social work that it needs to be accountable ... and that's from my past history in (another authority) where I just saw a mish mash response". This approach was supported by team managers in both authorities - "it draws more people into that process, more people can participate in the care management process"; "it would contribute to equity". This seemed to me to be a justification for a hybrid between the two roles, with the procedure serving the purpose of the exchange rather than the other way round. It will be very difficult for agencies to introduce this sort of model for care management, however, against the resistance of care managers who are suspicious of influences such as bureaucracy - "it's certainly a barrier (form-filling) between this relationship thing" - resource control - "in budgetary control terms what label do we put on the relationship? You can't cost it" - and other techniques of managerialism - "(targets) as a management tool, wonderful ... but in terms of dealing with clients as people it's not all that helpful ... it gives connotations of measurement ... and it doesn't matter what the quality of the work is".

Discretion versus Prescription

There were many examples of resistance to departmental procedures, with care managers using the phrase "we should do" this or "we ought to do" that. The *shoulds* and *oughts* revealed either an unwillingness, which, when challenged produced a grudging acknowledgement that they did, indeed, do it as intended, or, more interestingly, the revelation of a continued adherence to a method of working which was older, and more familiar - "If you ask my team manager I'm not supposed to have that role but I do it anyway"; "I'm actually doing very much the same thing as I always was". There was one example of workers in a team running two systems side by side - the old and the new - because they found the new system inimical to their preferred method of practice - "this is not policy, this is x's (team manager) own system".

This is evidence again of role confusion, but it also reveals the strength of adherence to traditional professional practices, as well as the degree of discretion care managers hold, despite the bureaucratic procedures. Care managers have the scope to resist policy intentions, and are doing so successfully, on this evidence. It was not confined to one agency, or to one profession. The corollary of this behaviour is that the baby of good practice is indiscriminately thrown out with the bath water of the new procedures.

One Shire manager spoke eloquently of the need for education in an academic sense, rather than training. Care managers, he believed, needed to have a deeper understanding of the changes of care management over traditional professional practice, so that they could really understand the advantages. This required a more academic approach to learning in his view, and suggested that going away to college was more likely to assist the process of reflection and adult learning than in-service training. We will return to this theme of the importance of reflection in the development of practice in later chapters. It was a central moment of learning and understanding for me.

Individual Care versus Community Care

Whether community care involves a process by which individuals receive their care needs, or is about the management of scarce resources on a more collective basis, takes us to the heart of the enterprise. It articulates the differences between care in the community versus community care, raised in an earlier chapter of the book. My over all conclusion from both Borough and Shire is that this is another issue which adds to the confusion about the role of care manager. Most are involved on a purely individual basis, assessing the needs of individuals and putting together packages of care to meet those needs. We will return to resource deficit recording later, but the resistance to this was most revealing. Most care managers can not see the priority for such activity, have little interest in strategic planning in general, and yet are very irritated by the lack of development of resources in some areas. The senior manager in Borough despaired of this lack of understanding and interest in structural influences on service delivery.

Care managers generally indicated that their prime responsibility is to the individual - "It's the individual we work with". Where there was a difference was in the way that care managers saw their clients within the broader community. There was good practice in networking and multi-disciplinary / inter-agency work revealed in both settings. It was particularly noticeable in Borough, with some good examples of people using networks, both formal and informal, to provide support for individuals. This was no surprise, perhaps, as these Borough workers were operating in small patches, where they had opportunities to get to know their communities and people within the community could get to know them. I was also impressed with the level of commitment, in Borough, to the importance of understanding the mix of culture within the patch. This was especially noticeable from the three black workers, all of whom mentioned the importance of ethnic monitoring, and all of whom noted the need for increased training in ethnically sensitive practice. There were white workers who expressed similar views in Borough, so this may be more an indication of agency ethos at work rather than individual perspective. Two white interviewees commented on how helpful it was to have colleagues from different ethnic backgrounds because their perspective was a dynamic force for the development of practice more generally within their team.

Acute versus Preventative Work

There was almost universal disappointment at the degree to which assessment practice involved patching up situations that had reached breakdown point before referral. Targeting those in greatest need was described as propping up the failures of informal care, and not good prioritisation - "if you don't do the preventative work, you're doing knee-jerk crisis work which is twice as expensive and half as effective". Putting resources into prevention was felt to be a far better way of working, but there was little opportunity for this. One Shire care manager mentioned a figure of 18% put aside for preventative work, but this was a vague allusion that could not be elaborated upon, and which did not crop up again. Such a policy certainly seemed to be undermined by the degree to which only the highest priority cases were being seen for assessment. Targeting those most in need is Government policy. The view of professional workers is that it is not a helpful way of achieving the over all aims of maintaining people in their own homes. Ironically, it was proving more difficult to resist this policy initiative than some of the others which might have a more beneficial affect on service users' lives.

Resource Constraints

Resource constraint was routinely quoted as the major stumbling block to the meeting of needs, although there was variation in this. Some respondents from both authorities said that the problem was not resources in terms of money, but of the availability of specialist service. When care managers were quizzed about this resource constraint issue, however, almost all of them owned that it was not a problem that they had encountered. They put this down to luck in their area, and predicted that things were likely to be much tougher next year. With continuing fiscal crisis, they may be so, although the evidence I collected suggests that the practice of most care managers in tailoring assessments to their knowledge of available resources may be more influential. Most admitted to this in both authorities, usually justifying this by an unwillingness to set up expectations with service users that they knew they could not deliver - "All my judgement is not to encourage people to hope for things which are not in the end going to be there"; "I have to say that if you do know that there are no respite places available to save your client distress and having raised hopes and then smashing them down, you don't recommend it".

This kind of pragmatism is understandable for staff who have to negotiate the complexity of relationships with vulnerable, needy and sometimes hostile people. The result undermines the practice of needs-led assessment. Assessment and care packaging in many of the cases that I heard about was driven by the care managers understanding of resource availability. Care managers, in addition, see very little worth in recording deficit - "there is a service deficit form we're supposed to fill in ... I don't, I haven't got time ... if it's something everybody knows I can't be bothered". These two practices combined, the resource lead to assessment and failure to record service deficit, result in central planks of policy for community care being eroded by care managers' practice. This is clear evidence of the distortion of policy intentions by street-level implementers.

When managers were asked about the likelihood of this occurring, those in Borough denied that it could happen and that all care managers understood the need to assess without considering resource availability - "I think I can confidently say that they are not influenced by the availability or unavailability of resources". In Shire some first line managers acknowledged what was happening and constantly reminded staff of the requirement that assessments should be needs-led. In Borough, care managers with first line management responsibility told of giving assessments back to workers to repeat because they were so evidently resource-led. Without a shift in attitude by care managers, possibly through the provision of opportunities to reflect upon the consequences of their actions and non-actions, this degree of exhortation is perhaps the only way to alter practice.

2. Use of Procedures and Resource Management

Allocation

All respondents were able to describe the system of allocation operating in their team coherently. Whilst systems were variable, there was a problem with the basis on which decisions were made. We will return to the variable use of agency priority systems below, but there was much evidence of the use of systems, designed to establish eligibility for service post-assessment, being employed to make decisions about allocation. This incongruence between procedure and practice was most apparent in Shire. The result was a danger of judgements about need being made prior to assessment. Such practice would undermine policy intentions. One middle manager in Shire expressed concern about the sophistication of decision-making in allocation. The procedure was believed to be too reliant on subjective judgements, and the hope was that more analytical methods, based on the priority matrix system could be developed - "people do need to learn a bit more about probabilities, making what are subjective, human emotional decisions but in a more analytical way". This desire for greater consistency is understandable. It needs to avoid prejudging priority of service delivery.

The Instruments of Assessment

These bureaucratic instruments were almost universally despised. The designers of these forms must be very thick-skinned individuals to cope with some of the venom directed their way from both care managers and first line managers. The accusation against those who design such forms was that they "only talk to computers", so perhaps they do not hear the complaints. I have already spoken of a few care managers, in both authorities, who found the prescription comforting, and others who felt that they combine flexibility with a consistency that is more likely to ensure equality of opportunity. When care managers were challenged on their negative attitudes to the forms many retracted their initial hostility as they found it hard to substantiate it beyond bare prejudice against bureaucratic procedures.

Some concerns remain, however, and many of them were offered by first line managers rather than their staff. The feeling that the forms were "computer-driven" and more useful for the quantification of assessment procedure was widespread - "it is computer-led and statistic and data-led, rather than practice-led"... Consequently first line managers readily admitted that they were of more help to them than their staff - "they do give me the answers I want if they are followed through". Even then, the kind of information available from the collected data was considered to be disappointing by most managers in both authorities. Managers felt that the quantitative data was crude and unhelpful, giving some weight to demands for more resources, but saying little about quality of work. Less assessments, they argued, may mean more effective assessments, and, therefore, less 'return' of service users, either as complainants, or in what is referred to in the health service as the 'revolving door'.

There was some articulation from managers and care managers in both agencies that the forms "get in the way of" the primary task of assessment, which is the formation of a relationship. One social work manager in Borough managed a team who felt de-skilled by the forms. She had instructed her staff not to think about the forms until after the assessment visit. The forms could then be filled in on their return to the office. This is another area in which policy seems to be unclear, because there was some belief amongst care managers in both authorities that they should complete the forms in the presence of the service user. This practice would maximise the likelihood of service user involvement in the process of assessment.

There would seem to be widespread belief, in conclusion, that the forms are there to serve the bureaucratic and resource control function of the agency. Even though this function is seen as valid, respondents felt that the forms should primarily serve practice needs as these are the ones most likely to affect the quality of service. As one manager said "a good assessment is not going to be a form-filling exercise". Dissatisfaction with the system leads to practice which undermines the good intentions of procedures, such as equality of opportunity, noted above.

Levels and Priorities

This is an area of some confusion, even where, as in Shire, there is a highly rational system of priority formulation, that has a substantial profile in the agency. Neither authority has a system of 'levels' of assessment, apparently. Some care managers said they did, but I understood this to be a confusion with the priority system. There was also confusion surrounding the use of a priority system in allocation as opposed to a priority system for determining service eligibility post-assessment. As far as levels of assessment are concerned, where the concept was understood, it was generally felt to be unhelpful. Once referred, all got "the complete works" as one manager put it. Indeed, there was much evidence of ad hoc arrangements for brief assessments, which did not mean that time resources were spent on "low priority assessments". I understood this to be against the policy of both authorities, but such was the diversity of views that it became impossible to be certain.

In Shire, as indicated, there is a 'high tech' system of priority formulation. It works very variably, according to the responses I received. It is used in a number of teams as a method of prioritising allocations, with priority scores being adapted after assessment, depending on the result. How it is used to establish eligibility is also variable. I understood that different areas should not have had different policies about which bandings will or will not receive a service, and under which circumstances, but, nevertheless, the practice varied both within and between areas.   Even given the attempt at rationality in prioritisation in Shire, managers admitted that it is a "fairly subjective score". The resultant scoring which can lead to service (or not) was seen as a "statutory obligation". As one manager put it "the Committee have said this is what Social Services will do, will offer assessment to anyone (with the right score), but obviously to make a score you have to do an assessment, so we are in a bit of a Catch 22".   A second Shire manager said "I think we are being advised to give everything that comes through the door a score". In recognising the "cart before the horse" nature of this advice, he went on to say that "a lot of the practices in the Department are quite idiosyncratic", with many people, in his view, having "their own ways of doing things". Another manager admitted that they write to some referred people refusing an assessment because they do not meet the criteria. This seems to be against agency policy as well as inequitable in the context of an ethos of needs-led assessment.   Both ethos and policy would suggest that no judgement should be made prior to an assessment.

One middle manager in Shire admitted that the latest policy on the system was unclear in her mind. Another was much more positive about the system and the way it gave practitioners protection from complaint, in that they could deflect complaints on to agency policy and away from personal decision-making. In order to do this care managers must be clear about what the latest policy is. In addition, the latest policy needs to be readily available to potential service users. In Borough, the system is far less prescriptive, so that the result is more flexibility, more imaginative use of resources, but the danger of less consistency, decisions being open to judicial review (only in Borough did I hear concern about this eventuality), and care managers feeling unsupported and open to complaints being directed at them.

Procedures and Equal Opportunities

There was quite a deal of evidence of care managers routinely and deliberately omitting to give copies of assessments and care plans to service users. Six care managers, between both authorities, stated that they do not routinely complete this task that some admitted was supposed to be mandatory. The reasons given were to do with user disinterest, or inability to understand, due to dementia or learning difficulty. One manager from Shire even claimed it was because users wanted to "save the trees". As implied above, it may well be the case that user's low expectations have resulted in a widespread display of apparent disinterest. Other care managers were clear about the need to give people their care plans and assessments, as of right, and felt that the onus was on them to explain why this was important.

My conclusion, on this evidence, is that there is probably a widespread belief amongst care managers that service users are not really interested in being involved in the process beyond giving information and receiving a service. The dangers of this leading to a practice that denies service users access to information that would be of use to them in making informed choices is worrying. It is another example of the opportunities practitioners have of using their discretion to undermine policy intentions.

3. Implementation of the Principles of Community Care

There are six areas, most already mentioned, that define the principles of community care policy. To what extent are these principles being undermined?

Service User Involvement

I have already said much about the widespread assumption that users are generally not interested in anything apart from getting a service to meet their needs. If this assumption continues, the intentions of a user-focus to assessment will not be realised and policy intentions will be undermined. It was interesting to go through the interview transcripts and note the replies to the question of who was involved in decision-making following an assessment. Only ten out of the 17 care managers said the user or the carer should be. That does not mean that they are not, of course. The point is, that when asked who should be involved in an assessment, user and carer did not immediately come to mind for a substantial proportion of care managers. The same point can be made for the general provision of information in relation to assessment and care packaging. The practice of providing information is very patchy in both authorities. Information provision is a key aspect of the care management cycle (Social Services Inspectorate 1991a, 1991b) and service users are less likely to be involved or enabled to make choices unless they are well informed.

The difficulties of being user-centred were honestly admitted by care managers in both authorities. It is much easier, when working with a user who has poor memory or severe learning disability to take over, particularly when they have no carer willing or able to assist - "you shouldn't do it (make assumptions about service user needs) but I think sometimes we do". Time constraints on care managers are considerable - "the reality is that you can't sit around and do it with them". Committed care managers admitted to being unable to sustain their anti-discriminatory practice under considerable time constraints - "we're not very good at sending the forms back for them to sign, it's time and pressure". The way this undermined morale and confidence was painful to see.

There was a commonly held belief that advocacy should be a role for care managers. Acting on users' behalf in trying to gain access to scarce resources, educating service users into the best ways to access services themselves, how to help users be more needs focused and less interested in actual services which may not meet needs for that individual were all believed to be important roles for care managers. Such was the level of role confusion, however, that many care managers were not sure whether agency policy allowed them to do this work or not. This, again was undermining of confidence.

The Relationship with Carers

Involvement of carers was generally at a higher level than with service users. One care manager was anxious about this aspect of her practice, recognising that it was time related but disempowering of the user. There was evidence from occupational therapists and some other care managers of a greater emphasis on listening to carers and not users - "I usually am much more comfortable in involving carers particularly as a lot of my clients have got a degree of mental impairment". Despite this, there was some evidence of imaginative practice with users to try and include them to the best of their ability, and recognition from at least one manager of the sophistication of practice necessary in resolving, or managing differences of opinion between user and carer, often where there was a substantial power imbalance between the two.

Choice and the Mixed Economy

Many of those interviewed revealed hostility towards the independent sector which was described as ideological - "I don't think you can trust the care of anybody, especially elderly people, to private concerns where they have to make a profit and they have to undercut". Others were dismissive of the quality of service offered - "they are so unsophisticated". There was also, however, concern expressed about the inflexibility of in-house Home Care Services. In this case independent sector agencies were seen as more responsive. There was little evidence of a burgeoning mixed economy of care services from these interviews. It was unclear, however, how sophisticated the information was that care managers were drawing upon. If such a knowledge base was not routinely developed, how can care managers know what is available within a mixed economy of care, across a formal and informal spectrum?

Community Care Plans and Strategic Planning

Community Care Plans were not mentioned as sources of knowledge for either practitioners, managers or service users, although they were intended by the legislation to be one of the forms of information provision that would improve services. Care managers are the eyes and ears of departments. Data collection for strategic decision-making will be much the poorer if care managers can not be persuaded that they have a part to play in this. Team managers in Shire and the senior manager in Borough felt that care managers need to be more actively involved. One manager said that failure to establish a clear role through a more academic approach to learning "makes it very difficult to get staff to identify service deficits ...as we get more money-led we need these deficits to show up and they are not". Care managers could be more involved by routinely being fed back information based on the collective data derived from their individual assessments. For this to happen they must be persuaded of the importance of deficit recording, as well as balancing needs-led assessment with unreal expectations. In this sense the future of implementation is in the hands of these street level implementers, and the degree to which they are to be encouraged to participate in rather than resist agency activities will be a key to successful implementation.

Financial Control and Service Delivery

Changes in accountability and flexible use of resources by people closest to users has been argued as a key way to provide needs-led services. Accountability and budgetary control has been largely decentralised in both agencies. Respondents enjoyed the opportunities to provide more imaginative and user-led services. This was, after all the negative versions mentioned above, an example of the existence of discretionary power which held the potential to develop policy according to intentions, rather than undermine it. Any loss of this discretion, it was believed, would result in a reduction in quality of service, particularly in the way that services responded to individual need.

Multi-Disciplinary and Inter-Agency Work

Most care managers are operating in a multi-disciplinary setting and feel happy to be so. There was some evidence of unease, however, particularly from recently qualified and unqualified staff. This seemed to be to do with perceived status, although, I felt that there was some concern that lack of role clarity left care managers vulnerable when working with, for example, health workers who were believed to have a clearer idea of their role. The senior manager in Borough expressed concern about the lack of confidence being displayed by care managers in this area of work. He believed that training was very important, and hoped that in-service training, as well as diploma in social work courses would address this area more. Occupational therapists in both authorities and care managers in Shire were less likely to reveal such concerns, and there was a fair deal of evidence, particularly amongst the more experienced practitioners that they felt comfortable and well-equipped to be practising within a multi-disciplinary setting.

Conclusions and Implications

The influences on care management practice in these two local authority social services departments are nothing like as clear as can be detected from reading guidance manuals and other local and central government documentation. When it comes to localised practice the tension between discretionary behaviour and prescriptive procedures finds care managers caught in a web of uncertainty. In these circumstances we find practices are inconsistent, roles are unclear, and opportunities for flexibility at its best and confusion at its worst, are rife. There is a professional agenda expressed by many care managers, and their managers. It is not a consistent discourse, however, and there is evidence of more than one professional agenda. I had described to me a more traditional practice which is individual based and problem focused. It is an approach which draws upon a medical model of disability, and is at odds with the more contemporary approach of user-centredness within the policy guidelines. There is also evidence of a very procedural approach, which borrows heavily from managerial interpretations of care management. Lastly there is a more contemporary care management practice which is informed by principles of user involvement, needs-led assessment, choice and empowerment. This practice is not exclusive to qualified social workers, although it is congruent with contemporary social work values (Banks 1995; CCETSW 1995).

These interviews would suggest that the procedures outlined in the Shire guidance manual and the Social Services Inspectorate document which serve as the principle source of procedural guidance for care managers in both authorities are 'more honoured in the breach'. The procedures provide a knowledge base for practice which has not been accepted by many care managers who are using their scope for discretion to undermine policy intentions. I have read many social services department care management guidelines and the Shire document is one of the better ones for clarity of practice and intent. It is very procedural, but does, as one Shire care manager said "describe good practice". Role confusion in care management is partly to do with resistance to what is seen as an alien culture by care managers. The definition of a client in the Shire Guidelines as 'someone on whom the Department is spending money' is the kind of 'value in action' that care managers resist. As one put it very prettily - "It makes my gorge rise".

This fieldwork indicates that social workers can make the shift in role and yet retain the fundamental tenets of contemporary social work values. Values are a crucial area for a complex reflective practice such as care management. Social workers are better educated for this approach to working with uncertainty, but the evidence suggests that the values of anti-discriminatory and anti-racist practice are seldom close to care managers thoughts when practising. Being user focused, being aware of the need to balance competing demands - e.g. of users and carers - and appreciating the effects of unrecognised power relationships are all crucial to the development of empowering practice, which most care managers expressed a commitment to. It is also a key aspect of community care policy.

There was little evidence of needs-led assessment. Resource availability, in both type and quantity, are the major influences on assessment practice. Care managers do not routinely record service deficits they come across. Being resource led, there is none to record. By over-reliance on carers for information, by assuming users are not interested in being involved and by not passing on documentation to them, care managers also fail to routinely involve service users in decisions that crucially effect their lives. These practices, if replicated in other social services departments, are undermining the intentions of government policy in community care.

The lack of interest and knowledge of agency and inter-agency procedures, especially in relation to service development and strategic planning, largely as a result of suspicion of senior management coupled with a focus on individualism in assessment and care planning, is also a great barrier to the success of the community care enterprise. This is again unfortunate, in that service development is going to be a key element if service users are going to be able to have anything other than Hobson's choice with regard to services. The result in relation to the particular needs of marginalised groups like black service users, will be very negative. Better communication between senior management and care managers through bureaucratic processes such as deficit recording and ethnic monitoring could hold the key to greater awareness and understanding, but only with a commitment to sharing information.

Targeting of resources on the most needy is not an efficient use of resources according to the evidence of these interviews. Engaging in mending broken informal support networks is also an ineffective way of maintaining vulnerable people's quality of life. Resources going into prevention and early identification would provide an effective role for care managers, increase morale, save money and provide services to improve quality of life. This would seem to be one of the areas in which care managers' critique of policy strikes a chord.

It is important to recall that I carried out these interviews in 1994. It might be expected that, one year into community care policy implementation, care managers would inevitably be struggling with these issues - trying to work out how to marry up their skills and knowledge with the expectations upon them. Whilst this is a valid perspective upon the findings from these interviews, there are two points that need to be made. Firstly Shire had made most of the substantive changes in relation to organisation and practice two years before implementation on April 1st 1993. Care managers in that authority had experienced the expectations of change over a long period and yet what they were telling me and what their colleagues in Borough were relating (in both positive and negative senses) was broadly the same. The second point was one that I was not to know at the time of my original analysis of the research interviews in this chapter. In the months after constructing this analysis, I presented these findings to groups of care managers who were carrying out very similar roles to those interviewed in Shire and Borough, at workshops in other local authorities. This occurred prior to the instigation of the co-operative inquiries described in chapter nine. There was admission from most of these participants that much of what I had learnt was still the case two and three years into implementation. With this explanation and hindsight, I am not convinced that all I was experiencing was teething problems with the implementation of a new policy.

I can only claim that this is my interpretation of practice within these two authorities. They all received a copy of the report I wrote for the agencies, upon which this chapter is based, but I received little validation of this despite asking participants for their views on my findings. A couple of first line managers replied that it was much as they expected, and the senior manager in Shire expressed irritation but not surprise by what I had learnt. The care managers, however, were silent. The validity of my learning is, therefore, suspect and this was an area for further exploration in itself.

The gap between expectations of practice from policy guidance and actual behaviour by care managers is, however, clear *from my interpretation*. I have documented the difficulties that care managers had in describing or analysing the origins of the knowledge that informs their practice. I have tried to convey some of the richness of their text in the way I have offered direct quotations. If that seems somewhat thin, then I believe that is a reflection of that struggle that many of them had in defining the knowledge base to their practice. Such reflection is not a routine activity for care managers even if it is considered widely in contemporary social work analysis to be fundamental to any notion of developmental social work (Gould and Taylor 1996). I was still left with not only the question of what knowledge base care managers do draw upon in analysing their practice, but also how they go about the process of making these connections. I was left, at this stage, then, with anomalies and puzzles that needed further explanation and exploration.

In my interpretation of the political agenda for community care, care management needs to combine a practice that is user-centred with one that considers resource constraints. This is the perennial problem for agencies, striking the balance between prescription and discretion. How does management enable skilled workers to demonstrate good practice, whilst remaining within resource constraints? How do you define procedures which enhance rather than stifle creativity and imagination? The tighter the managerial hold, the less flexibility, the more efficiency, the less effectiveness. Wherever the level is placed, however, rational policy making suggests the need for clarity amongst staff, with current policy readily available to both them and service users. In addressing the research questions, however, the opportunities for discretion leading to variable practice has proved to be considerable and there was evidence of respondents undermining procedural requirements and, therefore, policy. The question we are left with is whether this clarity that rationalist policy making requires is achievable or whether it is a phantasy. Chapter Four looks at this issue in the context of language and meaning. If clarity, or at least agreement between different stakeholders is impossible through rational top-down policy implementation, then implementation, through managerial practices and professional practices, as well as the methodological approaches to investigating these questions will need a different conceptual framework. Chapter Eight explores such a framework.

In conclusion, there is much to be done to bring the intentions of government policy more within the practice of key actors in the implementation process. Much of what could be achieved requires little in the way of new resources. The shift is more in terms of practice, and of the knowledge and understanding that creates meaning and informs practice by care managers, when carrying out the sophisticated practices necessary to fulfil their role. Clarity in defining that role is also a priority for care managers and their employing agencies. We need now to focus on answering the questions as to why this is happening and how an increase in that area of inquiry might lead to changes in practice across the board.

4 Key Texts that define Community Care

Introduction

This chapter looks at some of the key publications of the early years of Community Care policy implementation that define the context for care management in community care. The publications are all government or government sponsored documents which, we might believe, construct the reality of service delivery in community care. What are the expectations and intentions revealed in these key texts? It was important for me to address these questions more rigorously in the wake of the fieldwork interviews in Shire and Borough, because of the confusion of role which was so evident. Confusion of role was resulting in a haphazard use of discretion by care managers. The consequence of this ill-considered use of discretion was a fundamental undermining of policy intentions. To return to the key texts meant an opportunity to assess the degree to which policy and procedure intentions for care management were clear.

In this chapter I explore the theory of discourse, mediated by the concepts of actors and agency, arguing them as useful ways of making sense of government intentions in the context of community care legislation and policy. Whilst not the whole story, such an analytical approach does help address some fruitful questions as community care implementation continues to falter. What reality is constructed by the discourses revealed in these key texts? What relationship does this reality have to those involved in the negotiated process of service delivery in community care - service users and care managers? Is the voice of these constituents, which reveals their reality, one which can be heard within the competing discourses of community care? In analysing these texts, the chapter will describe the nature of the discourses revealed, and the conflictual relationship between them. Reflection on the implications of this struggle for practice forms the conclusions to the chapter.

We have noted already the degree to which the meaning of community care is contested, and that there is no consensus around the government's definition of this policy area.   The problem for policy implementation is to do with the way in which difference is *managed.* Giandomenico Majone (1989) speaks convincingly of the importance of 'evidence, argument and persuasion' for policy implementation in a democratic society. This chapter asks what forms of persuasive rhetoric are being used to define community care.

This line of argument takes us to the heart of many of the interesting debates in social welfare today. It helps to explain the tension between conflicting approaches to service delivery.   Much has been written about the degree to which professional, political and managerial agendas influence organisational processes both within community care (Pollitt 1993; James 1994; Brewster 1992) and more generally (Harrison and Pollitt 1992; Mintzberg 1989). The most difficult, but most pressing question remains how the voice of service users, who stand to gain or lose most in the battle for meaning, is going to be heard amidst these powerful alternative views.

Meaning, Knowledge and Power

Meaning, for social workers, is an important concept. One of the tenets of good practice is that social workers should strive to understand what service users mean when they describe their world. There are times when social workers have to impose their views, but they should always try to understand other people's meaning. The discussion here is not so much about the social work practice of understanding meaning, but does acknowledge that varying meanings and, therefore, views of reality, exist. These varieties of meaning are revealed through language, described, in its broadest sense, as *text*. In Derrida's oft quoted phrase - there is 'nothing outside of the text' (Parker 1992).

The concept of discourse tells us that knowledge is socially constructed (Rojek et al 1988).   A discourse that defines knowledge, although ephemeral, can be sustained, in a historical context, *for as long as people are prepared to believe in it.*   The concept used here, as in the Foucauldian tradition, is therefore to do with power - the power of one system of knowledge to define meaning and uphold one reality in the face of alternative versions. We have already noted that many learning difficulties (Souza 1997) and mental health service users have exposed assessment as an oppressive experience. It mirrors that of black service users (Watters 1996) who have spoken of their perspective and their culture being denied. The current experience is very far from the language of 'empowerment', or 'enabling choice', which is used to construct practice for assessment in the policy and care management guidance documents analysed below.

The Analysis of Discourse

Analysis of discourse may not provide the whole story, but it can be helpful in making sense of a complicated domain like community care. Charting the knowledge and 'coherent systems of meaning' (Parker 1992; p10) within key texts, both that which they immediately speak of and that which they connote (Parker 1992) or reveal through the use of metaphor (Soyland 1994), are important techniques of analysis. Derrida's phrase about 'text' provides the justification for looking at the documents listed below. The contention that 'language constructs the world' (Rojek et al 1988) is a useful starting point in analysing the relevant texts.

In as much as discourses objectify realities, it is the case that many objects do not exist outside of discourse (Rojek et al 1988). The success, then, of different discourses in speaking to us as subjects, is a key part of the analysis of the power of discourse. Does any particular discourse construct a reality in which we feel that we have a part (Rojek et al 1988)? The implications for social workers confronted by an unwanted management approach (Baldwin 1995), and service users with an unhelpful medical model (Ellis 1993; Morris 1993) need to be addressed if the aim of providing useful services is to be achieved.

It is important to reflect on the way in which service user or client is defined in these texts, as this influences the way subjectivity is created by the discourse. This form of objectification (Parker 1992) is exemplified by the process of attaching labels to people (Wood 1985; Lemert 1972; Becker 1963) so that they can be allocated services. The constraints on those things which people are able to speak of within a given discourse is an important aspect of the analytical technique (Parker 1992). An example of this is the use of professional language, the jargon that constructs a reality particularly for those people who understand the nuances of meaning within the discourse. Professional language does not only construct meaning in this sense but also restricts the boundaries of meaning. The medical model of disability for instance defines the individual person through their medical diagnosis. The difference between a medical and social model of disability came clear to me when, as a student I heard a social work colleague saying to someone 'he is spina bifida'. This is a constraint not only of what is deemed important, but also, what counts as permissable knowledge in the search for meaning in this person's life as they are being assessed for community care services.

This chapter will not use the analytical technique to dissect material as it is in other contexts (Stenson 1993; Burton and Carlen 1979). We are looking for evidence of discourse, and what that discourse might tell us of the different forms of knowledge that define the real worlds of community care.   This process involved choices by the author, and these are justified below.   It is necessary to 'persuade' (Soyland 1994; Majone 1989) the reader that there is merit in the interpretation of meaning within texts.

Discourse, Agency and Actors

Discourse does not just define reality, it defines the context (historical, political and economic) in which the discourse can exist, and the extent of its influence over action (discursive practices). Foucault noted the ways in which meanings are 'embodied in technical processes, in institutions, in patterns for general behaviour' (Foucault 1977, in Macdonell 1986). It is not knowledge of technologies, or techniques in themselves which define intervention. It is rather 'knowledge we have about the human capacity to apply them' (De Vries 1992). Techniques of intervention and institutions, like discourse itself are socially constructed and defined by negotiations over time. A social services department, its policies, procedures and staff practices are not determined, but negotiated, within the context of competing discourses.

There are dangers within these arguments, of a reification of discourse (Burman and Parker 1993). It is not a deterministic model and the potential for negotiation of realities is always present.   An actor oriented approach which recognises the existence of 'multiple realities' (Long and Long 1992) and the process of negotiation of a joint creation of knowledge can ensure that there is no slide into assumptions about permanence or absoluteness.   There is evidence from research both from within (Lipsky 1980; Baldwin 1995) and beyond (Long and Long 1992; De Vries 1992) the social work arena to indicate that practitioners understand the potential for agency, and develop, through negotiation with other key actors, including service users, techniques for protecting their scope for discretion. It is also a helpful analytical tool when investigating the use of discretion by social work practitioners. To what degree, we must ask, are social workers aware of their scope for discretion and to what extent do they self-regulate their use of agency? We look more at this experiential arena in later chapters. Agency, as a concept, is helpful in arguing against the more deterministic usage of discourse. Reality is negotiated through interaction and agency, not exclusively determined by discourse, or ideology.

Choice of these Texts

The first criterion in choosing 'key texts' was that they should all be closely related to Government intentions. There is an assumption, therefore, that the White Paper (D of H 1989) and its associated Policy Guidance (D of H 1990), Audit Commission Reports, Social Services Inspectorate (SSI) Guidelines and Department of Health (D of H) sponsored documents have the approval of Government in their publication.

The White Paper and its Policy Guidance choose themselves. This *is* Government policy for community care to all intents and purposes. As attempts to explain what the Government means by these key concepts of assessment and case (later changed to care) management introduced in the White Paper, the SSI documents are essential to analyse. The SSI, D of H sponsored document which takes these concepts further (Smale et al 1993) is more problematic. Its sponsorship by the D of H puts it into contention as a key text. It is because it is the one government associated document that attempts to analyse concepts introduced in other texts and to treat them as more than given which makes it important to analyse.

The influence of the Audit Commission (Henwood 1992; Malin 1994) on the monitoring and development of Government policy is not contested. The problem is the choice of text. It might have been others, such as 'Making a Reality of Community care' (Audit Commission 1986), the persuasive arguments of which was largely responsible for forcing the Government to reduce public expenditure on private residential care and launch the move towards legislation which began with the Griffiths' Report (Griffiths 1988). Whilst the development of a historical perspective is of interest, this chapter will explore an Audit Commission view closer to the time of policy implementation.

Analysis of the Texts

Caring for People - The White Paper - and Policy Guidance (D of H 1989; D of H 1990).

It is hardly surprising that a White Paper employs political rhetoric. The Paper lays out Government Policy, and they will want to give it the hard sell. So what might we believe that the Government's wishes are in relation to community care?

The White Paper outlines six key objectives (D of H 1989; p5). People will in the future be enabled to 'live in their own homes'. Assessment will 'always take into account the needs of caring family...'. 'Individual needs and preferences' will be the proper stuff of assessment. Social Services will 'enable' a 'flourishing independent sector', meaning 'private and voluntary providers'. The responsibilities of agencies will be clear enough so as to 'make it easier to hold them to account'. The final objective is to 'secure better value for tax payers' money'.

The White Paper declares reassuringly that '...ability to pay does not and should not in any way influence decisions on the services to be provided.' (D of H 1989; p28) It is in this context, and when the Policy Guidance is studied, that the rhetoric about choice and good quality care begins to unravel. The new funding system gives Local Authorities the 'responsibility for managing this budget and making best use of funds available in the light of an assessment of an individual's needs' (D of H 1989; p 64). 'Budgets...' as the Policy Guidance points out (D of H 1990; p6) '...have never been unlimited.' The balancing act of maintaining 'best quality care' within limited budgets is acknowledged. What is not spelt out is that such a policy will narrow the band of service users who are 'targeted' as being 'those people whose need for them (services) is greatest.' (D of H 1989; p5) This narrowness of eligibility is far from the political rhetoric of high quality services for people in need.

In practice, therefore, a framework for rationing decisions has to be constructed. What is revealed about the Government's expectations about such a framework? The way in which the political rhetoric is compromised throughout the Policy Guidance undermines intended outcome. The construction of subjects, people in need, and the way they are objectified, labelled and lumped together (not only those in 'greatest need', but also those falling into particular categories - '*the* elderly' or '*the* disabled'), also conflicts with the concept of individual choice.

The same rhetoric is there in the Policy Guidance concerning 'partnership and collaboration' (D of H 1989; p14) and 'providing individual choice and self determination' (D of H 1989; p23). The problem with these words is the context in which they are set. Thus care management systems should 'concentrate on those with greatest needs' and in planning community care services, all agencies will 'need to determine their objectives and priorities within resources available.' (D of H 1989; p24) 'Equal opportunities for all' is a metaphor. It says 'for all', but it connotes select groupings of people 'in greatest need.'

This context reveals the 'coherent system of meaning' (Parker 1992; p10) that we are searching for. 'Individual choice and self determination' (D of H 1990; p23) sound like phrases from professional social work discourse (CCETSW 1995), but the meaning of these concepts is revealed by the phrase 'within resources available'. The latter phrase is more powerful knowledge because it defines and limits. 'Choice' is expansive and unlimited. In addition, resources are defined and restricted by Government decree. The discourse of resource control (which I will refer to as managerial discourse), is a powerful body of knowledge that defines the meaning of community care in the White Paper and Policy Guidance. It has determined a particular set of practices and institutions within the organisation of community care. Most Social Services Departments separate purchase from the provision of care, all are required to have community care Plans that reveal relevant priority needs and the resources available to meet them, and the techniques of prioritisation - assessment and eligibility criteria. These are the discursive practices of the managerialist discourse.

To deconstruct statements in this text is to reveal fundamental contradictions in Government policy. Care plans must meet user's needs but they must be cost effective (not cost too much). They must meet user's needs, but user's and carer's preferences are only to be 'taken into account' (D of H 1990). These contradictions are managed through the certainty of the dominant discourse, the resource control functions, priorities, targeting, and eligibility criteria. Choice within resource control is a very particular and limiting version of the word choice. It actually means constraint. Choice equals constraint. How can the 'voice' of service users be heard in this context?

The implementation of these processes requires a process of negotiation. The managerialist discourse, as revealed in this text, is the context in which actors will negotiate with other actors - colleagues from their own and other organisations, as well as service recipients - in order to create a world of community care. The managerialist discourse is a powerful force, it defines a particular knowledge and meaning, connotes particular discursive practices and institutional arrangements, but outcome is a product of negotiation within a context of competing discourse.

Evaluation of community care implementation rarely considers the tension between opposing discourses, and seldom acknowledges the scope for discretion by workers. Where it does, (Baldwin 1995) there is evidence that agency, when aggregated (it is far from clear that such discretion is being applied collectively and deliberately by care managers) can undermine intended outcomes whether it is defined in managerial or political terms. It is in this fashion that social workers, as care managers, can act as 'street level bureaucrats'. This is the term that Lipsky (1980) developed which is analysed in detail in the next chapter.

The Audit Commission Text

The Audit Commission is not averse to using political rhetoric to frame content. On page one of The Community Revolution (Audit Commission 1992) the text declares that 'the first aim is to empower the service users and their carers giving them choices...' On page 18 it is noted that 'demand for community care services is always likely to outstrip supply.' By page 20 problems of implementation are being laid at the door of unacceptable management systems. The necessity of a mixed economy of care, targeted services, separation of commissioning and providing, flexible operational style and staff training are quoted as the keys to required change. The certainty of these systems in achieving the desired outcome is not in doubt.

Shortly after this (Audit Commission 1992; p35) the Report insists that 'what is meant by need must be rigorously defined.'   'The definition...', the Commission continues, 'depends on an authority's priorities for support and the people it intends to target, which in turn depends, in part, on the resources available.' Need, in itself a complex and contested arena (Doyal and Gough 1991), is to be defined by Local Authorities' policy guidance and determined by the level of resources available, not the voice of individual need.

This report has much to say about the skills of care management. The list of desirable qualities in the mock advertisement (Audit Commission 1992; p39) is another example of doublespeak. Attributes such as 'the ability to listen... be non judgmental... gain the trust and confidence of users and carers... be imaginative...' is translated in the body of the text in managerial terms. 'Care Managers must become skilled at using financial systems and information technology', make 'hard practical decisions on service provision' and be able to 'negotiate with providers, influence the contract-making process and commission local providers' (Audit Commission 1992; p39).

There is, in this text, a separation between the rhetoric and the practical application of technique in managing the policy changes. So, for instance, on page 45 the text lists the 'norms and criteria against which quality outcomes and effectiveness can be measured.' These include consultation with users and carers. This is not congruent with the suggestions for managing budgetary controls made on the preceding page. Here the 'accuracy of budgets can be improved by a careful review of past performance, the setting of clear priorities, enforcement of cash limits and careful costing of new initiatives.' This concern for accuracy reveals the language of control and costing. There is nothing here about choice or needs. 'Accuracy' is a metaphor for control. This kind of discourse places the Audit Commission's version of community care into Foucault's discipline thesis. It undermines professional discretion and pollutes the fertile soil of 'voice'.

There are other ways in which this text undermines the meaning of consultation with service users. Collaboration, particularly with the NHS, is seen in terms of 'needs goals and priorities, resources, assessment and care management models, information requirements, criteria for service eligibility and evaluation for quality.' (Audit Commission 1992; p.54) These are the discursive practices of managerially defined partnership. Collaboration with service users, in stark contrast, is conceived of in terms of surveys and 'locally arranged meetings in community centres and village halls'.

This Report provides substantial support to the managerialist discourse within the White Paper and Policy Guidance (D of H 1989, 1990). The same coherent system of meaning is revealed. Community care is about establishing a framework for the distribution of scarce resources. Social relationships are objectified to a greater degree than in the White Paper. 'Target groups' are defined organisationally (managerially) before the techniques of prioritisation are applied to actual people. In this way subjects who might become service recipients are created as objects of interest within the managerialist discourse.

The techniques of managerialism - the discursive practices - are also developed in a more sophisticated way. Assessment processes, eligibility criteria, quality outcomes and effectiveness criteria are all defined within the meaning of the discourse. The coherence of the discursive practice with the discourse itself makes this text a good example of Foucault's contention that there is no separation between theory and practice. There is little room for alternative versions within the all-embracing combination of knowledge, power and action.

Social Services Inspectorate Texts

The SSI documents employ forms of knowledge from competing discourses, and present a confusion of meaning. Social Services Departments have drawn heavily on these texts for their guidance documents. How far care managers have been able to establish a coherent role for themselves is an important question for the implementation of the community care changes and was an area of great concern revealed within the research interviews analysed in the previous chapter. The texts now analysed provide nothing clearer in the way of an answer.

1. Summary of Practice Guidance

This summary attempts a definition of terms. A model of care management is described followed by a brief analysis of the concept of need. Given the vastness of the literature (Doyal and Gough 1991) which deals with this concept, to attempt the definition in just over one page is courageous. What the text does say about need, however, is significant. Needs are defined as the 'requirements of individuals to enable them to achieve, maintain or restore an acceptable level of social independence or quality of life, as defined by the particular care agency or authority' (SSI 1991a). Staring such terms as 'acceptable', 'independence' and 'quality' full in the face, the guidance places the onus of definition on to Local Authorities. This exposes the emptiness of the political rhetoric that community care is concerned with user-defined needs and choice of service.

The Summary speaks the language of user-led services when discussing 'tailoring services to need' (SSI 1991a; p.16), 'developing commitment to individual Care planning' (SSI 1991a; p.16), 'promoting wider choice (SSI 1991a; p.17), and 'meeting the needs of disadvantaged individuals more effectively' (SSI 1991a; p19). This is congruent with the political rhetoric of the White Paper. When it comes to organisational arrangements, however, other considerations are revealed. One of the more subtle pieces of conjuring in community care implementation has been to define the purchaser / provider split as enabling a needs-led focus to assessment for services. That this is the method of introducing market forces into welfare service provision is a meaning only revealed through the persuasive, metaphorical use of words such as 'choice' and 'mixed economy of care'.

Attention is paid to a professional discourse in this Summary. 'Assessment that seeks to define individual need' is seen as calling for a 'higher level of expertise'(SSI 1991a;p.22). This, plus the discussion of needs discussed above, the definition of shared values on page 25, and the high priority given to training in anti-discriminatory practice (SSI 1991a; p.29) are indicators of a professional (particularly social work) agenda.

There is a problem, in analysing this text, in looking for coherence of meaning. The knowledge revealed, which defines the world of meaning for care management is confusing. This Summary of Practice Guidance is attempting to give all-comers something to work upon. This is more problematic when we compare the Managers' and Practitioners' Guides.

2. Practitioners' Guide

It is not surprising that this Guide speaks the language of professional social work. An interest in moving beyond presenting problems is revealed in Stage 2 when practitioners are urged to 'be alert to indications of more deep seated or progressive difficulties' (SSI 1991b; p40). Social work claims an interest in holistic assessment, and the guidance argues the virtue of comprehensive assessments that enable 'individuals to be considered as a whole, enhancing the prospect of an integrated response to their needs' (SSI 1991b; p48).

Identification of 'the strengths as well as the weaknesses of individuals' (SSI 1991b; p50) is seen as good practice. This is almost a direct quotation from the statement of requirements for qualifying social workers produced by the validating body for social work education - the Central Council for Education and Training in Social Work (CCETSW 1995), and also places the guidance in the professional camp. Communication skills are central to the practice of promoting participation. Relationship is a key concept within professional social work discourse, and it is given a central role in the process of assessing need in care management (SSI 1991b; p.52) .

Whilst the professional agenda may be to the fore, there are elements of managerialism. Assessment of need is established within agency defined boundaries. Part of the care manager's role is to implement these definitions in practice. 'Practitioners must decide on the eligibility of users for assistance from their own agency.' (SSI 1991b; p.53) Despite the emphasis on user and carer's priorities, care managers are informed that 'the priorities of users will then have to be matched against those of the authority or agency' (SSI 1991b; P.54).

The elements of managerialism within this text, are tempered by the over all meaning revealed. The objects referred to by the text are within professional social work discourse. The word 'users' has been taken in preference to 'clients', but they are the same people, constructed within traditional professional discourse. Users are defined through the relationship formulated as part of the social work process of assessment. It is a traditional model of professionalism, with the emphasis on the technique of the practitioner. The use of professional language constrains the realm of knowledge and meaning within this document. Even the references to ethnic and cultural difference are defined in the context of professional technique, and not of rights. The correct course of practice will, so the connotation goes, achieve the desired outcome. There is a scientific rationalism reflecting a discourse of certainty that reveals an interesting congruence between managerialist and traditional social work discourses. When the document speaks of 'enabling individuals', looking at 'strengths as well as weaknesses', when it stresses the importance of 'communication' and 'relationship', these words and phrases have resonance for social workers within their traditional knowledge base, and give them clues to the ways in which they should behave.

3. Managers' Guide

The Managers' Guide attempts to present a coherent package of care management, with organisational, inter-organisational and training implications. As text it speaks the language of more than one discourse. The knowledge base is, however, managerialist.

Choice is a word that cuts across discourse but is most noticeably prevalent in the political rhetoric of community care. So the separation of assessment from provision will give 'access to a wider range of services'

(SSI 1991a; p.35). Unlike the Practitioners' Guide, however, this text goes further, talking of the need to 'establish a market situation in which assessing staff are able to choose' (SSI 1991a; p.36). Staff are encouraged to be more 'entrepreneurial'. This language indicates that not only is it the market which is seen to provide the best result for choice, but it is staff who choose and not service users. This is a notable deviation from previous use of the term choice when it was presented within the domain of service users . In this context it is not an issue of needs, let alone rights, but one of practice. The 'correct' organisational structure - 'a market situation' - will enable the member of staff to adopt the best approach, which is described as 'entrepreneurial'. This language can be directly differentiated from the language of professional practice in the Practitioners' Guide. Being 'entrepreneurial' does not validate practice within a social worker's traditional knowledge base. It is a phrase that jars with the language of enabling. To be an entrepreneur is to be more interventionist than to be an enabler. The two words come from different cultures, the first from the world of business management and the second from social work. The first is evidence of managerialist discourse, the second of a professional social work discourse. They are both, however, similar, in that they connote a certainty that rational practice will produce consistent results. This use of rationalism from both professional social work and managerialist quarters is an area of theoretical analysis that is returned to in Chapter Eight.

This text is full of the language of managerialism (Pollitt 1993) and audit-speak (Power 1994). Once an agency has defined the needs that it will meet it is urged to make 'relevant and *cost effective* use of available resources' (SSI 1991a; p.46; original emphasis). Quality standards should be 'accessible to measurement' for the purpose, amongst other things, of staff performance measurement. A check back to the Practitioners' Guide reveals that, in this text, quality standards are not related to the assessment of practitioners' performance but to meeting the needs of service users. The same language, in a different context, reveals a different meaning and constructs a different social world. Care managers when asked to pay heed to developing quality standards (a noble aspiration on the face of it) may well suspect that it is a management device and, therefore, understand the phrase to mean measuring their performance. The increasing prevalence of the concept 'performance related pay' is likely to close the circle of their scepticism. Such scepticism can lead directly into the kind of sabotaging of policy intentions described in the previous chapter.

This whole document attempts to balance the need to control staff (and therefore the allocation of resources) with the need to allow the use of discretion (to free up the entrepreneurs who will develop flexible services). This a classic problem for public sector management (Pollitt 1993). The ambiguity displayed means that the document fails to portray a coherent and consistent role for care managers. On page 50 (SSI 1991a;) the need for balance between 'regulation' and 'discretion' is noted to encourage 'accountability and equity' on the one hand and 'autonomy and flexibility' on the other.

These concerns expose an interest in the needs of public service professionals, but they are concerns of management. The language, and the discourse revealed is managerialist. Quality of care has to be quantified so that it can be measured. This approach removes the concept of quality from the sophistication of social work practice, and from the need to balance risk and empower users to make real choices in their lives. Quality becomes an organisational process defining an 'artificially constructed environment of action' (Jackson 1991).

It may be that there is something disingenuous about this critique. Perhaps we should not be surprised that a Managers' Guide is informed by managerialism. But there is an issue of power here. Power to define the reality of welfare service organisation. The success of this discourse in influencing practice is likely to have a substantial effect on outcomes. The theoretical concept of power within discourse suggests that each power base holds its own contradiction. In the case of care management, this means that practitioners have an opportunity to be autonomous actors, performing with 'agency' (Long and Long 1992), negotiating the rules and regulations laid down by organisations, whatever discourse they might be informed by. This is not just a theoretical concept. Lipsky (1980) describes a similar process. Policy is not what is written in agency documents, but the practice of 'street level bureaucrats'.

4. Empowerment, Assessment, Care Management and the Skilled Worker (Smale et al 1993)

This text, whilst acknowledging political rhetoric, is rooted in professionalism. But this professionalism is not a traditional social work discourse. It uses the language of 'relationship', 'empathy', and 'communication', but sets it in the context of user involvement (Morris

1995). When it speaks of bureaucratic procedures they are related to equality of opportunity, and not resource control for its own sake.

Three models for assessment are defined - Questioning, Procedural and Exchange. 'In the questioning model the professional is assumed to be the expert in identifying need' (Smale et al 1993; p.7). This is a traditional model of professional discourse - assessment as judgement based on forms of knowledge restricted to those qualified to practice. There is little place for the service user as the expert in their own experience. 'In the procedural model ... it is assumed that the managers drawing up guidelines for workers have expertise in setting the criteria for resource allocation' (Smale et al 1993; p7). This model of assessment is informed by managerial discourse, utilising a scientific rational approach to organisational considerations.

It is in the exchange model, in which 'all have equally valid perceptions of the problems' (Smale et al 1993; p.7) that a new model for practice resulting from 'redefining professional expertise' (Smale et al 1993; p.13) is conceived. We can now look at a few examples of this non-traditional professional discourse. It provides us with a notably different perspective on community care, which sits uneasily alongside the managerial rhetoric of the Audit Commission text and Managers' Guide, as it does with the more traditional approaches to professional practice revealed in the above texts. This approach suggests that different world views will be revealed through assessment. Assessment is then less a process of applying known techniques, whether they be informed by traditional professional or managerial discourse, and more a practice of making sense within a context of contested meaning.

The Exchange model is about using relationship to communicate understanding, often across cultural divides, to create a climate of participation for all involved in making sense of problems and searching for possible remedies, either within service users' own strengths, or from external resources. Thus people 'come together and arrive at a mutual understanding of the nature of the problem' (Smale et al 1993; p.11). Professional expertise is identified as 'facilitating people's attempts to articulate' their own needs, with 'sensitivity to ... cultural ... differences'(Smale et al 1993; p.13), whilst recognising the 'patterns of relationships that precipitate and perpetuate social problems' (Smale et al 1993; p14). Among the tasks of such a professional are the ability to 'facilitate full participation', make a 'holistic assessment', and 'help create and maintain the flexible set of human relationships that make up a "package of care"'(Smale et al 1993; p.45).

Even where the language of managerialism is employed, it occurs in a context of this new professional orientation, and is redefined by it. 'Holding and using a budget' and 'gate-keeping goods and services' (Smale et al 1993; p.45) are 'not ends in themselves. They are tools for helping people work together...'(Smale et al 1993; p.45). Even the purchaser / provider split is re-framed in this way. This split takes on a different meaning when it is defined in terms of relationships rather than the reification of 'packages of care', and 'when the currency is not money, and the transaction is the communication of different people's perceptions of their needs, their feelings and their choices over how their care, that is their set of crucial relationships, is to be organised and maintained' (Smale et al 1993; p.58).

Conclusions

In reading the key documents listed it seems that there are agendas being set out which, using our theoretical model, can be described as discourses. There is a managerial discourse (Pollitt 1993; James 1994) revealed in most of the above texts, in particular the Audit Commission reports and the Managers' Guide. This agenda is informed by a market economy discourse, but also reveals a model for the control of those assessing need for services. This model is particularly sophisticated because it is presented in a context of devolution of financial control to the lowest point in the system. Care managers should note that another aspect of the managerialist agenda is quality control, through targets and performance indicators which cast a strait jacket around the shoulders of managers despite their budget-holding responsibilities. The domination of the managerialist discourse severely restricts the possibility for other forms of knowledge to inform practice. If performance is defined by the measurement of numbers of needy people targeted, rather than informal care networks sustained, then preventative work is effectively programmed out of professional practice.

Professionalism provides a second discourse, most notably espoused in the Practitioners' Guide. Professional discourse is revealed through an interest in the use of relationship for the purposes of 'exploration' with service users, through concentration on the importance of creativity in a practice for which the individual worker has a personal/professional responsibility (as opposed to an agency/professional responsibility). Skills in communication and multi-disciplinary work, amongst others, are the techniques, or discursive practices of professionalism. We can also see, especially in the NISW document, the beginnings of a different, and more contemporary professional discourse which takes professionalism beyond the constraints of traditional approaches and their rationalist certainties.

Also revealed in these texts, and particularly in the White Paper, is a political rhetoric designed to sell the policy as the only way of understanding 'Community Care in the next Decade and Beyond' (D of H 1989). This political rhetoric is sophisticated because it steals the clothes of other agendas in making its case. There is a nod towards the professional lobby (particularly the professional social work lobby) in much of the literature which recognises that there are people, mainly social workers, who will be involved in the implementation of policy. Managerialism is a key aspect of the political rhetoric because of the resource constraint imperative.

Political rhetoric also speaks the language of service user involvement. In one sense it seems that this is what it is about - choice and quality services to meet the needs of individual service users. Local Authorities are even exhorted to take into consideration the needs of black and minority ethnic communities. Up until recently this consideration has been noticeably absent in government rhetoric. Whilst the concept of user involvement reveals a different meaning within the competing discourses, it holds the potential to deconstruct, and, therefore, redefine traditional managerialist and professional discourses.

Managerialism, with its power base within government and senior management in many local authorities appears to be the most powerful discourse. But power, as Foucault and Derrida have argued (Boyne 1990), is not such a simple concept. Discourses do not either have or not have the power to determine outcomes. It is a process of negotiation, with practitioners carrying out assessments having substantial opportunities to influence outcomes, using their discretion to define policy as what Lipsky (Lipsky 1980) termed 'street level bureaucrats'. Care managers also have opportunities to influence outcome through the empowering potential of partnership with service users. Recording unmet need, for instance, is one managerialist practice that holds the potential to deconstruct managerialist power. Sadly, care managers seem loathe to engage in the practice (Baldwin 1995; Sadd 1996) as we have noted in the previous chapter.

There is being waged, in social welfare agencies, a battle of competing discourse, conflicting meaning, but there are other fields of conflict that also have bearing on the outcome.   The undermining of the professional qualification of social work through changed job descriptions, and, more particularly, the relentless shift to competency based qualifications, are more likely to undermine the professional discourse, particularly the new professionalism revealed in the Exchange model of assessment (Smale et al 1993) and elsewhere (Bamford 1990).

Reflective practice is one of the fundamental aspects of the Diploma in Social Work, which is still a generic qualification requiring holders to be able to transfer their understanding and skills from setting to setting.   National Vocational Qualifications, that use validation of practice as the sole method of assessment, hold an inherent danger of apprenticeship - training people for a defined job. This approach to training is more in tune with the scientific rationality of the managerialist discourse.   The reflective practice of the contemporary professional discourse involves an acknowledgement of uncertainty not compatible with managerialism.   It is important to note that it is far easier to wield power from a position of certainty. With the persuasiveness of 'evidence-based practice' in LASSDs proving on the ascendance in recent times, there is now a further string to the bow of positivist certainty as it determines organisation and practice within community care.

But are community care assessments like that? Does assessment subscribe to the notion of certainty within managerialist discourse, or are there more complex processes involved? Assessment practice can be defined as a process of negotiating uncertainty with, and giving voice to, vulnerable people, often across cultural divides. To impose the certainties of scientific rational managerialism is doomed to failure if the intentions of community care are to meet expressed need and provide choice from a developing and flexible mixed economy of care. In a context of rationing scarce resources, however, managerialism's rational and certain approach is the one beacon of light in a thoroughly murky world. We need to ask whether the clarity of the managerialist agenda is a sustainable reality. Or should we accept the inevitability of murkiness and try and ensure that those people who have to negotiate a way through it are fully equipped to make the journey?

The analysis of policy intentions within this chapter has persuaded me that a unified linear approach to a complex process such as the implementation of community care policy is unhelpful as both a source of explanation and as a basis to guidelines for practice. Contradiction and discontinuity of meaning revealed through discourse analysis is helpful in making sense of the evidence of implementation deficit revealed in the activities of street level implementers in Chapter Three. If this analysis undermines the certainties that we may have about community care as a major policy area - and the way care managers' practice can add to this undermining of policy intentions only increases this understanding - we need to ask what are the implications for policy implementation? If the reality of community care is going to be the result of negotiations between key actors in a context of powerful and competing forms of knowledge, then perhaps it might be more helpful if this process is acknowledged in organisational structures. Policy implementation could then be constructed through co-operative participation between politicians, managers, practitioners and service users. Social work assessments would be constructed through a genuine 'partnership' between professionals and service users and research outcomes would be constructed through collaboration between researchers and those traditionally treated as the objects of research, as were the care managers in the first phase of fieldwork interviews. Having revealed this contradiction I felt that it was important to explore the possibilities for a different epistemology and methodology which would be more helpful for both explanation and practice. These are areas of investigation that are now explored from a theoretical analysis in the next part of the book. They raise questions which were addressed in the second stage of empirical work and which will be looked at in the final two chapters.

5   Lipsky and Street Level Bureaucrats - a Source of Explanation

Introduction

We have already looked at policy implementation theory in chapter two above, focusing some attention on the distinction between top down and bottom up approaches.   Concerns about rationalism in top down approaches to implementation have been aired, although it is acknowledged that rationalist explanations still hold considerable influence on the discursive practices of policy implementation. The point here is not to dismiss top down explanations because that would be to dismiss what is normative practice. The difficulty with rationalism is that it claims that problems of implementation imposed from above can be overcome given the correct conditions for implementation. This claim for a regulatory form of implementation is built upon an epistemology of scientific rationalism which is less sustainable if it can be shown that there are other factors that skew 'perfect' implementation, and over which rationalist practices such as traditional managerialism have little influence. It is at odds with other explanations which suggest that professional discretion in decision-making has some effect on implementation.   This chapter provides such theoretical evidence, and is thus congruent with the empirical evidence presented in chapter three. Rationalism would also be undermined if it could be demonstrated that, within a 'rights' approach to policy implementation there is evidence that citizen involvement might have some effect that influences the implementation process. This is not the brief for this book, but opens up a fascinating area for fruitful future research.   In the previous chapter the concept of discourse, actors and agency was addressed. It was seen how an analysis of discourse in the key texts for Community Care exposes the confusion of policy intentions and helps explain the implementation deficit that results from role confusion among key street level implementers. This was the same role confusion noted in the interviews in chapter three.

The focus of this book is on the former of these two challenges to rationalism in policy implementation - that is the role of practitioners in creating policy through their practice. We need, therefore to look at Michael Lipsky's concept of Street Level Bureaucrats and see to what extent that helps explain the findings from the research interviews analysed in the previous chapter. The chapter will also look at other studies in which the effect of discretionary behaviour is analysed. It has been noted that there is a lack of research in this area (Goodsell 1981) and, even though that was alleged some 16 years ago, it is still a claim that is remarkably true.

The justification for this chapter's focus upon the role of the front-line or street-level policy implementer follows from the empirical work analysed within chapter three. From my interpretation of the interviews carried out in that chapter, and from supporting literature (e.g. Ellis 1993), it has been seen that there is apparent evidence of street level workers undermining policy intentions. What theoretical explanations are there for this state of affairs? I need to look at Lipsky and present a critical analysis of those parts of his book which help me in my search for an explanation, but I also need to address the whole concept of discretion and its use in organisations such as Social Services Departments which are responsible for implementing community care policy. In the latter stages of this chapter I use the most helpful aspects of the Lipsky formulation to revisit the activities of the care managers of Borough and Shire to make further sense of not only what I understood to be happening there, but also, and more importantly, to start thinking of ways in which the negative outcomes of such practices could be altered.

Discretion in Public Policy Implementation

There is a great deal of discussion about the existence and role of discretion in the literature about policy implementation and organisational analysis (Bamford 1989; Clarke et al 1994; Hill 1997a; Hill 1997b; Hogwood and Gunn 1984; Hugman 1991; Pressman and Widavsky 1973). None of these authors, providing a range of attitudes and analysis to the theme of discretion denies its existence, although it is true to say that most have a very negative view of the effects of discretion. The rationalists, such as Hogwood and Gunn, are keen that their formulation for rationalist top-down implementation, looked at in more detail in chapter two, would reduce the negative effects of discretion. Most of the other authors seem rather to accept its inevitability within complex bureaucratic organisations.

But what is discretion and how is it practised? Two versions of the concept are important to stress. Firstly there is discretion as the interpretation of rules within complex organisational procedures. Secondly there is discretion as the departure from rules or rule-breaking. In this version front-line workers (in the focus of this book) use their scope for autonomy to act in a way that is outside of either the statutory authority that defines the limits of their activities (illegal) or the rules - policy and procedures - of their employing organisation (ultra vires). This tension between rules and discretion is an argument around legitimacy, democracy and accountability (Hill 1997b). This takes the argument into the arena of power relationships, although I am going to restrict such discussion to noting that the activities of front-line workers, when they use their discretion, is an example of the exercise of power. Within our focus of attention (care manager practice in the assessment of vulnerable adults) such exercise of power has the potential to severely affect the life chances of people who are often already marginalised through the social processes of disability, age and gender discrimination and racism. In chapter seven we will note how the "combating" of such processes is a core value of social work practice.

What are the origins of this discretion? The inevitability of discretion in organisations such as Social Services Departments is argued as a result of the complexities of policy, organisation and practice. The policy process which takes implementation from consultation to white paper, through statute to policy guidelines and government department circulars, to local government policy and procedure and implementation through managerial systems is one of great complexity. There is no straight line from statute to front-line implementer and this degree of complexity leaves opportunities for interpretation through available autonomy by all those involved along the way. There is, then, the potential for the policy framework to be moulded into different shapes and forms. I have already described an aspect of this process in chapter four in which the SSI guidelines on care management for managers and practitioners (SSI 1991a; SSI 1991b) provide two substantially different versions of how care management can be interpreted (the managers' guide and the practitioners' guide).

The second point about the origins of discretion concerns the nature of the decision-making within the practice in question. The greater the degree of decisional complexity involved, the more likely discretion will exist in both its rule-breaking and rule interpretation formulations. Assessment of the needs of potential social services users is argued as a prime example of this sort of decisional complexity.

The last question about discretion that I need to focus upon before moving on to look more closely at Lipsky, is about the outcomes of discretion. It has already been pointed out that most analyses of discretion in public policy seem to have a more or less negative articulation of its place within the policy process. The normative distinction that is made is the degree to which discretion is more or less *structured*. The degree of structure allows for greater or lesser degrees of *control* of discretion by the upper echelons of bureaucratic or managerial structures within organisations, without any expectation of removing it as part of the process.

Another distinction recognises that discretion can fall somewhere between the unacknowledged habits of routine practice (even within very complex tasks), as we shall see Lipsky suggesting, and the very deliberate and considered use of reflection upon degrees of autonomy in the process of decision-making. At this stage I only wish to note that this is a continuum of the use of discretion that is not endorsed in the literature. I will return to it as a continuing theme in the remainder of the book as I believe it takes us into an analysis of discretion that holds far more positive opportunities than most observers allow. Discretion can, therefore, be more or less reflected upon by those who exercise it with (or without) those in management positions who have responsibility for the control of front-line staff. Outcomes, at the former end of this spectrum, could theoretically involve the use of discretion as a positive part of front-line practitioners' work as they engage collaboratively with other stakeholders in the process of policy implementation. It is this kind of analysis that may get us beyond the tried and failed approaches to discretion which have involved either attempting to control it through autocratic managerial means or to structure it through technocratic organisational processes. Both are rationalist expectations which have, as I argue, been notably unsuccessful in reducing the negative effects of discretion on policy implementation.

Michael Lipsky and Street Level Bureaucrats

'I argue that the decisions of street level bureaucrats, the routines they establish and the devices they invent to cope with uncertainties and work pressures, effectively become the public policies they carry out' (Lipsky 1980; p. xii). This is the exposition of one very influential and persuasive version of the bottom up approach to policy implementation. Hudson in his analysis of Lipsky's theory adds that - 'If we wish to understand policy implementation we must understand the street level bureaucrat' (Hudson 1989: p. 397).

It is not the intention, in this chapter, nor is it feasible within this book, to offer a complete analysis of Lipsky's work on the origins, context and outcomes of discretion as practised by street level bureaucrats. What follows is a synopsis of those aspects of his book which are most helpful as I try and make sense of the part played by street level policy implementers as they engage in the use of their scope for autonomy as I observed it in the empirical work of chapter three. Lipsky looks in greater detail than this chapter would warrant at the organisational context of street level bureaucratic practices. Much of this material is of less relevance to this book as it reflects organisational structures from a different welfare bureaucracy (the United States) and in a different era (the 1970s). There is much that is different in the United Kingdom system in the late 1990s, most notably the introduction, since 1979, of the "marketisation" of social welfare services and of managerial systems that have undermined more traditional administrative bureaucracies that dominated social welfare organisation prior to the Conservative government that came to power in 1979. In addition, although he does address fiscal crisis and resource shortfalls, this context is now even more acute as a result of a number of dynamic factors including heightened client expectations following the development of notions of citizen's charters, and demographic changes (notably an increasingly ageing population - one of the great successes of the welfare state).

As I say, Lipsky was writing in the late 1970s, producing a theoretical work offering an explanation of the practices of public sector workers in the United States of America. It is an analysis which uses a very eclectic theoretical approach (Hudson 1989), but which draws upon extensive empirical work carried out in the United States within a number of public sector organisations employing a range of semi-professional workers, including social workers.

Lipsky claims that, in response to organisational and workload pressures, street level bureaucrats (who included social workers in his analysis) develop working practices which maximise their use of discretion. Procedures are adapted to the client or service user and the service user is adapted to the procedures. In this way street level bureaucrats construct a version of the service user that is easiest for them to deal with in the midst of their workload pressures. This results in 'client processing' (Lipsky 1980 p. 25) in which 'routinised responses' socially construct clients. He argues that 'client characteristics do not exist outside of the (bureaucratic) process that gives rise to them' (Lipsky 1980 p.59). Street Level Bureaucrats practice at the interface between those (desperately) seeking services and the scarce resources that constitute those services. They thus hold considerable power, through the interpretation of policy guidelines and organisational procedures, to decide who passes through that interface and who does not. The power to decide and define is what Lipsky addresses as street level bureaucrats' professional discretion.

Discretion is, then, a key concept for Lipsky, and he argues its origins in much the same ways as I have addressed above. As Hill (1993c) maintains in his analysis of Lipsky's book, discretion has its source in four different areas:

- deliberate recognition of local autonomy
- failure to resolve political dilemmas which lead to ambiguity
- the problems of prescribing standards
- limitations placed on the regulation of practices (Hill 1993c: p.88).

Lipsky's argument is that street level bureaucrats 'characteristically work in jobs with conflicting and ambiguous goals' (Lipsky 1980: p.40) which results in the inevitability of discretion. Lipsky is very exercised by the gap between the *intentions* of street level bureaucrats as they attempt to do a 'good job' (Lipsky 1980: p. 82) within their personal set of values, and the outcomes which actually undermine those values. The context of practice that Lipsky describes - resource shortfall, indeterminate objectives and a dearth in controls on the use of discretion - describes an organisational environment that has changed little since his book was published in 1980, apart from a worsening of the resource position because of demographic changes and political decisions.

Lipsky describes a vicious circle in which the behaviour of street level bureaucrats undermines their own estimation of the value of their practice. This threat to the purpose of their role damages their morale and reduces their confidence in a way that reinforces the negative behaviour and completes the circle. Later on Lipsky argues that it is easy to change the policy but less easy to change such behaviour which he claims is 'rooted in survival' (Lipsky 1980: p. 187). This behaviour is exemplified by discretionary practices which he argues result in modifications to practice in three different ways.

1. *Modifications in practice that 'tend to limit demand'* (Lipsky 1980: p.83) come as a result of street level bureaucrats using their powerful position to informally ration access to resources. The use of labelling and stereotyping of clients pigeonholes people into those who receive a service and those who do not.

2. *Modifications in 'their concepts of their jobs'* (Lipsky 1980: p.83) result in street level bureaucrats accepting limitations and redefining their practice to make day to day work achievable.

3. *Modifications of 'their concepts of clients'* (Lipsky 1980: p.83) happen in a number of ways. One example would be the creaming off of clients thought most likely to succeed and be reflected in outcome returns (a specialist team accepting referrals of reduced complexity and increased likelihood of success rate would be an example). Another would be 'worker bias' (Lipsky 1980: p.107) including racism and prejudice, and the creation of informal categories of deserving and undeserving clients whose cases would subsequently be given weighted priority.

This, effectively, is the problem of unbridled Street Level Bureaucrat discretion as Lipsky describes it. As with other writers (Ransom and Stewart 1994; Ham and Hill 1993) Lipsky's stance is that discretion is inevitable in a bureaucracy. In pondering how discretion might be controlled and made a more positive dynamic, Lipsky looks at the operation of accountability. He looks at this concept in four forms:

1. Accountability, Proceduralism, Supervision and the Control of Discretion

This is the bureaucratic arena which has, in contemporary local authorities, been heavily dominated by managerial techniques (Clarke et al 1994; Pollitt 1993; James 1994). Different forms of management will result in different outcomes. Is management, notably through supervision, a form of support and development for practitioners, or a form of control? If there is an element of control within supervision, is it delivered through opportunities for reflection and guidance, or is it more coercive, with sanctions for failure to follow prescribed courses of action? In support of Lipsky's arguments around accountability and procedures Pottage and Evans (1994) have argued that practitioners are caught in a 'gap between expectation and ability to provide' (Pottage and Evans 1994: p. 12), and that, as a result, accountability is met through the imposition of procedures in increasingly inflexible form. The imposition of accountability on practitioners by management, through procedures, is maybe an understandable response when certainty and predictability is the holy grail to be sought, but the lesson from Lipsky is that resistance through the application of discretionary behaviour is still available to street level bureaucrats.

2. Accountability, Consumerism and the Control of Discretion

Consumerism is a now a powerful discourse determining procedures which may influence the discretionary powers of Street Level Bureaucrats more than during Lipsky's era. Both "new right" versions and those built upon a rights discourse, however, place limits upon the use of discretion.

3. Accountability, Legislation, Complaints and the Control of Discretion

Accountability in this case provides legal and procedural sanctions and opportunities for service users to challenge the actions of local authorities and their employees. Some of the well publicised judicial review cases, such as those in Gloucestershire and Avon, are good examples of service users making use of legal redress to reframe a local authority's discretionary powers as legal duties.

4. Accountability, Professionalism and the Control of Discretion

This is another area where there has been a shift in conceptualisation, this time in relation to professionalism. New professionalism (Bamford 1989; Hugman 1991) which recognises the rights approach to service delivery, which works from a social model of disability (Oliver 1996) and views service users as equal citizens, will affect the manner in which discretion is used. Advocacy and user-centred practice would be more prevalent than the worker-driven and service orientated approach that Lipsky described.

It is Lipsky's contention that coercive forms of management will result in covert, and therefore, unbridled or unreflective forms of discretion which are likely to be destructive of policy intentions. It is this apparent determinism - coercion leading to unconsidered use of discretion - that has led some (DeVries 1992) to label Lipsky a behaviourist. His argument about the behaviour of street level bureaucrats would seem, however, to be informed not by a positivist epistemology such as behaviourism, and to be more in the social constructivist, phenomenological, arena (Hudson 1989). Lipsky's evidence points towards street level bureaucrats acting with agency in the way, for instance, they construct clients through client processing. This evidence is supported by that in chapter three. Social workers as street level implementers operate in a context which persuades them to act in certain ways, as a result of the power of rhetorical devices such as the discursive practices of managerialism, but they do act with agency, constructing a social reality, in relationship with others, for themselves and their clients, which effectively creates social policy at the street level. The use of discretion by street level bureaucrats as defined by Lipsky is more than just poor practice. In his book, such practice actually constructs policy. The problem, for policy implementation, is the ill-considered and unreflective way in which Lipsky claims this will habitually happen. Buffeted by the alternative discourse of rationalist implementation procedures and scientific managerialism, street level bureaucrats resist. There is, then, a separation between espoused theory and what Argyris and Schon have called 'theory-in-use' (Argyris and Schon 1996: p. 14). Practitioners' espoused theory and theory-in-use, the latter of which will very often be tacit and not explicit, will, according to Argyris and Schon, very often be incongruent. It is this difference that is fundamental to Lipsky's arguments about the use of discretion, although the Argyris/Schon book continues by arguing that the accumulation of theory-in-use in an organisation, again very often different to that espoused by organisational policy, 'largely accounts for its identity over time' (Argyris and Schon 1996: p. 14). This is another, and slightly different version of the street level bureaucrat theme, in which collective action constructs not just policy but organisational identity as well. Chapter three's evidence again supports this contention. The result is a skewing of policy intentions and the loss of opportunities for harnessing available knowledge skills and values to a developmental practice which would enhance the quality of service provided.

The focus here is still upon the very negative connotations of discretionary behaviour, and this is compounded within the other views that I am now going to look at. It is important that we acknowledge the argument that it is in the nature of working in the public sector that there is such demand from below and such expectations from above that it is almost impossible for street level bureaucrats to manage their day-to-day workload except by engaging in the use and abuse of organisational processes and procedures in the self-protective way described. The interpretation of procedures in what I argue is an ill-considered or unreflective use of discretion will offer them some protection from the buffeting of demands, will construct policy over time, and will alter practice in a way that takes them away from the notion of public service and social justice that very often propelled them into their job in the first place. I have already indicated the evidence of the way this gap undermines morale in chapter three. As the rest of this book unfolds, however, there is an argument for a differential perspective upon discretion which argues that there are opportunities for a more positive and developmental practice of discretion that would construct a less gloomy view of policy implementation than that espoused so far.

Other Views of the Practitioner Role in the Policy Process

Not only is there a surprising lack of empirical research into the effects of practitioner activity, and notably the use of discretion, on policy implementation, but also there is very little in the way of critique of the Lipsky book (Hudson 1989), even from rationalists who favour the top down approach to explaining policy processes. There is a critique of the focus on clients and officials as the key players in the policy process which argues that acceptance of this as the status quo would undermine democratic processes in policy implementation. It is claimed that enhanced citizen control in particular would lead to the 'fragmentation of political control of the bureaucracy' (Mladenka 1981; p. 158), and that this will undermine the democratic process in local government should it be allowed to continue in unbridled form.   Since this time, of course, the whole conceptual area of citizenship has shifted considerably and contemporary approaches to citizen control, whether from a new right consumerist perspective or a rights approach both have considerably more weight as acceptable and persuasive forms of rhetoric in the policy process than they did in the early eighties.   There still remain the arguments between representative and participative forms of democracy, but it is more difficult now to argue persuasively that democracy was under threat from citizen involvement.

Clarence Stone's analysis looks at 'attitudinal tendencies among officials' and asks why there has been so little impact by what he terms 'client-oriented workers' (Stone 1981; p.63) on quality of service. This is an attempt to look at the effect practitioners can have on service quality. He recognises political and resource constraints as factors which takes his analysis outside of the main thrust of Lipsky's argument. In addition he notes the way in which administrative structures and managerial strategies impose restrictions on the development of good practice in facilitating citizen involvement in service delivery.   In criticising 'blind faith in management from the top down' (Stone 1981; p.64) Stone seems to express a greater faith in the ability of practitioners, working within managerial structures that do not equate with control, to deliver a better quality of service.   Lipsky charts the difficulties resulting from the unbridled use of discretion. Stone notes the positive effects that can come from a more positive approach. This is a theme that will be picked up again in the conclusions to this book.

Hasenfeld and Steinmetz (1981) investigated   'client-official encounters in social service agencies', adopting exchange relationship as the theoretical explanation. This is interesting in as much as it brings in the resource rationing aspect of such encounters and thus the power relationships involved in these transactions to a far greater degree than the Lipsky book allows. In describing the tactics used by officials to tackle clients, however, the list is similar to Lipsky's. Thus they describe the manipulation of waiting lists, 'status degradation' (Lipsky 1980: p. 90) which is effectively stigmatisation, 'discourse control' (Lipsky 1980: p.90), the control of conversation through the use of powerful professional language, and labelling, which they refer to as the reification of staff bias - 'the power to label is the power to determine outcomes' (Lipsky 1980:

p.91). This does not undermine the Lipsky book, rather enhances his approach by a more sophisticated analysis of power relationships. Their recognition of miscommunication through the failure to deal effectively with cultural differences brings their analysis into the contemporary arena as far as understanding about anti-discriminatory practices in social work are concerned (Baldwin M 1996b).

The Hasenfeld and Steinmetz analysis is also interesting and takes us beyond Lipsky in as much as they address the other side of official - client exchanges. They accept, and then list, the ways in which, despite power differences, clients can influence encounters. Although most of these tactics are defensive and, therefore, negative in consequence, it is interesting to get a beginning idea of the possibilities for constructing policy outcomes through exchanges between clients and officials. Bureaucrats, then, are not the only people at the street level to be influencing policy outcomes. Evidence from the field of development studies (Long and Long 1992; De Vries 1992) already quoted in chapter 4, presents a sophisticated analysis of the ways in which the "clients" of non-governmental organisations in developing countries engage in a process of constructing policy outcomes through relationship and exchange with fieldworkers. The Hasenfeld/Steinmetz book is supported by this approach.

Hall's empirical study of the influence of receptionists in determining practice outcomes (Hall 1974) in social services departments takes us away from the use of discretion by professional practitioners, but, nevertheless, reaches conclusions which support much of the Lipsky book. Starting from a desire to analyse the processes of decision-making in resource allocation, Hall allowed himself to become side-tracked into what is a seminal study of organisational processes in social welfare agencies. He was interested in the use of discretion in decision-making, noting that 'some rationing methods are obvious and are made explicit by the service providers. Others are less obvious, implicit and frequently not even recognised for what they are' (Hall 1974: p.17).

The list of tactics is again familiar. Manipulation of eligibility criteria, stigmatisation and personal predilection of service providers are some examples of the ways in which staff, aided by the activities of receptionists, used their discretion with the result that policy intentions were skewed. Hall diverges from our prevailing thesis at least to some degree, in that he advocates 'rational decision-making' (Hall 1974: p.18) as the answer to this unbridled use of discretion. Hall acknowledges the basic problem by noting that formulation of policy is one thing 'but of at least equal importance is our understanding of the techniques and administrative problems of translating policy decisions into action' (Hall 1974: p.37). Whilst Hall recognises the distortion of policy through discretionary behaviour as a valid explanation for policy deficit, he appears to adopt a more rationalist view as far as answers are concerned. In acknowledging the problems of curbing discretion and thus reducing job-satisfaction for staff, he ends up asking more questions than he answers.

The other study that looks at the behaviour of street level practitioners comes from a similar period in the development of UK social welfare organisation, and, usefully, focuses on the behaviour of social workers. Carole Satyamurti's study of 'Occupational Survival' (1981) is also a seminal work, providing us with an insight into the behaviour of street level bureaucrats, from a differing theoretical perspective to that of Lipsky's but coming to some similar conclusions. She starts with an intention to study the 'strategies that social workers adopt, individually and collectively, in order to make their work tolerable to themselves. As with the Hasenfeld/Steinmetz study, Satyamurti adopts an interactional analysis, although focusing principally on the practitioner side of the exchange. She lists some of the survival techniques used, such as 'boundary maintenance' (Satyamurti 1981: p.134) in which clients become to a large extent 'social products ... generated in interaction with colleagues' (Satyamurti 1981: p.139). This process results in the stereotyping of clients through the imposition of clinical and moral frames of reference which effectively construct clients as deserving or undeserving. These 'modes of classification' were used 'to extend their area of autonomy and protection' (Satyamurti 1981: p. 136).

There is no doubt that Satyamurti's analysis constitutes a blistering attack on social work practice in that era. She gained the impression that 'the need for social workers to survive the contact with the client was more pressing than the occupational goal of effectiveness in solving a client's problem' (Satyamurti 1981: p.139). Whilst Satyamurti notes a probable 'gap being experienced between an ideal way of working and what can be achieved in practice' (Satyamurti 1981: p.181) she allows herself little opportunity for compassion towards her subjects. I was reminded first of David Brandon's (Brandon and Jordan 1979) definition of suffering within Zen philosophy as the gap between expectation and experience and secondly was interested to note the echoes with my own interviews, recorded in chapter 3, and in which I was concerned greatly about the effect that the employment of the tactics that reveal this gap will have for morale amongst practitioners, with all the implications for quality of service.

Satyamurti includes a useful and interesting analysis of the 'interplay between aspects of the structural and organisational situation in which social workers were placed, and their subjective experience of, and response to it' (Satyamurti 1981: p.180). This is an area which we need to focus upon carefully and which is largely ignored by Lipsky, and dismissed by rationalist approaches to policy studies. In human services such as social work this interplay will always and inevitably exist. Ignoring it, in the way that rationalist approaches do (this may be why Lipsky's failure to address this has lead some analysts to refer mistakenly to his as a behaviourist approach (De Vries 1992)), means that the consequences of the interplay are not dealt with. These consequences listed by both Lipsky and Satyamurti are crucial to understanding the concept of implementation deficit and argue strongly for an interactionist and constructivist approach to the analysis of policy implementation. This, in turn will lead this argument to conclude that positive and constructive acceptance of the networks of relationships involved in the policy process through increasingly participative forms of organisation between all stakeholders is likely to enhance the implementation of policy as intended and reduce the degree of negative use of discretion and consequent implementation deficit.

The 'attempts to maximise autonomy' noted by Satyamurti are similar to some of those noted by Lipsky and have echoes from the interviews carried out with care managers analysed in chapter 3, where, it will be remembered, some care managers were, as an example, using priority criteria that long pre-dated that introduced by the authority for use in the implementation of the new community care policy. Limitations in the work process, including role confusion, for instance between themselves and officers from other agencies, and the confusion between care and control as forms of practice, as well as bureaucratic controls all led to the adoption of defensive practices. In addition, the nature of social services departments as residual organisations in which responsibility was not clearly delineated, and responsibility and legitimation for activities was therefore blurred, all allowed practitioners to construct their own defensive tactics which constituted a divergence not only from policy but also, in Satyamurti's analysis, from reasonable and humane practice. 'Evasion of bureaucratic requirements' (Satyamurti 1981: p.187) was thus rife in the practices she observed.

Satyamurti's conclusions are to note the poor practice that results from the unbridled use of discretion but also the failures, for individual, collective and organisational reasons of a more co-operative and participative approach to occupational survival that might result in more favourable service delivery.

Empirical Evidence from Work with Social Workers and Care Managers

How is discretion within welfare bureaucracies operating in the contemporary era? Lipsky's structure is a useful way of looking again at the analysis of interviews with care managers, detailed above and elsewhere (Baldwin 1995 and 1996a). This research reveals evidence of Lipsky's contention that social workers act as Street Level Bureaucrats in developing their own behaviours to deal with problems experienced in organisational structure and workload management. This was happening routinely in each of the three ways that Lipsky describes.

1. 'Modification in Client Demand'

There was much evidence of care managers undermining one of the central parts of Government policy - the development of responsive services (D of H 1989). The practice techniques for this which are described in the policy and practice guidance (SSI 1991 a & b) are needs-led assessments, recording of unmet need and a user-focused (participative) approach.

Most care managers interviewed in the research spoke of tailoring assessments to resources known to be available in order to avoid raising expectations for service users. Consequently few of them recorded unmet need. This is partly because all needs are met if assessments are tailored in the way described, and partly because care managers lacked faith that recording deficit would develop resources.

There was also a widespread belief that service users do not want to be involved in the assessment process, as long as they get a service. There are problems in carrying out needs-led, user-focused assessments where there are communication difficulties (service users who have learning difficulties or dementia for instance). This seemed to be used routinely as an excuse to deny service users an opportunity to participate in procedures that fundamentally affected their life chances.

It is worth noting here that the most influential contemporary theory of need (Doyal and Gough 1991) argues strongly that one of the two basic needs required as a precursor to meeting intermediate needs, is autonomy. If care managers who are supposed to be "needs-led" are routinely denying people that basic need for autonomy by reducing their opportunities for participation in processes that affect their life chances, then they cannot, in the Doyal and Gough conception, be meeting the needs of vulnerable members of society who are potential service users.

2. Modification of Job Conception

There was some evidence of care managers accepting the limitations of a bureaucratic approach to assessment and care management, but the more typical response was one of resistance. Forms - the instruments of bureaucracy - were believed to undermine professional practice, and to block the formation of positive relationships from which assessment and service provision flow. The forms were also viewed as a symbol of organisational interest in quantity not quality of practice. In other words the triumph of a rational managerial system over professional concerns.

There was also a lack of role clarity revealed, with practitioners within the same teams (let alone the same authority) revealing different use of procedures. This is perhaps not surprising given the ambiguity around policy guidance (Baldwin 1997). The point here is the way that people behave when their role is unclear (and stressful by its own nature). There was evidence of confidence undermined, inconsistent practice and, in many cases, a rejection of new procedures in favour of old and familiar routines.

3. Modification of Client Conception

Whilst care managers found it hard to articulate the value base to their practice, there was no evidence of the discriminatory approaches that Lipsky describes. There was no cream-skimming, stereotyping or dividing the deserving from the undeserving by individual care managers. Labelling, which Lipsky also identifies as a typical Street Level Bureaucrat procedure, is an organisational routine within contemporary Social Services Departments in which no one gets a service until they are fitted into a user category. It is not so much a sin of individual care management practice at the street level - it is what they are required to do by procedural dictate.

There was some evidence of unconsidered assumptions about what clients are like, particularly in contrast to carers. There was a belief, for instance, that carers are more articulate in defining the needs of service users, and this became another justification for a non-participatory practice. This is a modification from policy in which service users are defined as self-determining, to one in which "they don't want to be involved". Racism, as a form of prejudice identified by Lipsky, was not obvious. Indeed there was some evidence of very effective anti-racist practice. It seems there has been some development in this area since the 1970s.

The interviews analysed in chapter three provide support for Lipsky's contention that unbridled or ill-considered discretion results in not just a distortion of policy intentions but the creation of policy outcomes which are at odds with those intentions. We have here evidence of the eternal tension between prescription and discretion. How does management enable skilled workers to develop "good" practice whilst remaining within policy and practice guidelines, many of which are intended to manage scarce resources? There was evidence of a neo-Taylorist (Pollitt 1993; Clarke et al 1994) approach to management, rationalising practice into prescribed courses of action. This approach is being resisted by care managers who were behaving in a number of Street Level Bureaucrat-type ways. The interviews, therefore, provide evidence of resistance to implementation which result in unintended policy outcomes. The fieldwork evidence concludes, therefore, that a) it is right that Street Level Bureaucrats can skew implementation and b) that because of this, rationalist implementation theory that seeks to suggest that policy can be imposed from above in the way intended is unhelpful as both explanation and method because of the inevitability of discretion (Ransom and Stewart 1994; Ham and Hill 1993). We remain with the question as to whether, or to what degree, such discretionary behaviour might be harnessed to policy intentions, and what measures would have to be taken, what organisational procedures would have to be in place, in order to maximise the positive over the negative employment of discretion. We need to take a closer look at some of the practice theory, for both management and professional practice, and explore the degree to which it helps explain the problems that remain with policy implementation. This is where we now move on to in the following two chapters.

6 Management and Managerialism

Introduction

The purpose of this Chapter is to analyse the knowledge base and assumptions of public sector management which are likely to affect policy implementation. When I speak of management in this chapter, I mean public sector management, even though many of the versions of management within the public sector have drawn heavily from private sector practice and theory. Whilst the private sector may have provided much of the influence, there is a richness within social policy and public sector management literature which has supplied the main sources of analysis and, therefore, offered the primary sources of knowledge as we try and make sense of the phenomenon of management within contemporary community care organisation. The chapter will look at the degree of congruence between forms of knowledge for management and for policy implementation already looked at in previous chapters.

In the next chapter I will do the same for social work theory. We can note that scientific rationalist forms of knowledge construct a powerful social reality which has a substantial influence on both the practices and theories that inform them in the field of community care implementation. In other words there are traditional forms of theory and practice in both management and social work which are informed by a scientific rationalist epistemology and positivist philosophy, as there are in policy implementation theory. They are deterministic, functionalist and claim to pursue truth through the certainty of their technique. It is interesting then to note the degree to which there is a clash between management and professional practice, for example as noted in chapter three. People whose actions are informed by either, even within their similar paradigm are, as we have seen from the research interviews, inherently suspicious of the other. Even if they both pursue certainty in a similar way, it would seem perhaps the versions of certainty are somehow different. A closer look at this clash of culture (James 1994: Harrison and Pollitt 1994) is required. It is important to explore why there is such incongruence as it is likely to fuel the problems already noted about the unbridled and unreflective use of discretion by street level bureaucrats.

The certainties of dominant forms of knowledge are being increasingly challenged by alternative, contemporary views within both management and social work, as indeed they are within policy implementation theory (Warde 1994; Schram 1993; Fischer 1993; Dobuzinskis 1992). On the face of it we could assume that these new ways of constructing management and social work practice, which are more attuned to the uncertainties within human behaviours and are more prepared to understand the ways in which realities are socially constructed through relationships rather than fixed and 'out there', might be mutually supporting. This book concludes with consideration of the circumstances in which 'new managerialism' and contemporary social work knowledge might co-exist in a way that would be developmental for policy intentions.

Management Theory and the Influence of Managerialism

Management has been argued as an essentially modernist activity - 'the application of formal logic to the solution of problems' (Carter and Jackson 1993). How sustainable is this view, which effectively lumps together a broad range of management models which reflect an equally broad spectrum of theoretical perspectives? The implication in the Carter/Jackson view, which is very dismissive of this managerial world view, is that all managerial approaches are doomed to failure within a postmodernist perspective. We need to test this out by looking carefully at analyses of management theory in practice in the public services, and contrasting more traditional approaches (often referred to as 'Taylorist' or 'Fordist') with more contemporary approaches such as the Human Relations School, Total Quality Management (Morgan and Murgatroyd 1994) and learning organisations (Mintzberg 1989; Senge 1990; Argyris and Schon 1996).

It is important to look at management because it has not only assumed a high status within the development of social care, but also because many interviewees quoted in chapter three were inherently suspicious or even hostile to management influence. This suspicion is supported by other analyses of the public sector. Ann James, for instance, notes that 'the emergence of managerialism has, it seems, all too often been at the expense of the professional.' (James 1994; p.30)

Whilst James speaks of the emergence of managerialism, this should not be taken to imply that it was an accidental or organic development. Management was quite deliberately introduced into traditional welfare bureaucracies by the Conservative Government in the 1980s and 1990s. Although there was more control over this introduction within the Civil Service through the Financial Management Initiative and Next Steps (Pollitt 1990; Flynn 1990), and within the National Health Service, nevertheless the introduction of managerialism into local government organisations such as Social Services Departments, was heavily influenced by both Government activity, and by that of its close allies such as the Audit Commission. The organisational imperative of the NHS and Community Care Act is a managerialist approach. We have already seen in chapter four the extent to which the Social Services Inspectorate guidance on the introduction of care management is influenced by managerialism, and it is arguable that the introduction of Community Care policy was an attempt to introduce managerialism into adult social welfare services (Clarke, Cochrane and McLaughlin 1994).

What this deliberate move was trying to replace was Weberian type welfare bureaucracies which, within new right analysis, were believed to stifle efficiency and waste resources. The introduction of management would have many benefits for a Government with a particular ideology to pursue. It would undermine local authorities which were seen to be dominated by high spending Labour controlled Councils, it would cut back on the total public sector budget, and curb the power of professionals who were perceived as being a block to the development of the more efficient processes of the market in welfare distribution (Clarke 1995). The construction of what has been termed a 'quasi-market' (LeGrand and Bartlett 1993) was the aim of the introduction of managerialism into local government. Creating the environment for the successful implementation of the manager's right to manage has been a powerful rhetoric in the 1980s and 1990s. There was also the associated issue of political control of local government. Managerialism is argued by many commentators as an attempt to achieve political control over bureaucracy within public services, notably local authorities in our case example of community care (Walsh 1995; Clarke 1995; Farnham and Horton 1993; Clarke, Cochrane and McLaughlin 1994). There is an interesting tension here around legitimation and accountability that it is important to note in preview of later discussions around service user involvement and participation. The 'right to manage' which was such a powerful form of rhetoric in Conservative Government approaches to the public sector, is at odds with other approaches to legitimation and accountability. Citizenship as a concept, in its consumer guise, does pose some problems for the right of the manager in this sense, but not to the degree that citizenship from a rights perspective (Taylor et al 1992) challenges this approach. In addition the right to manage has also set up a considerable tension with the more traditional form of accountability within local government, that is representative democracy. So whose rights are paramount when it comes to the organisation of community care? Is it the elected representatives, the managers or citizens, either as consumers within a welfare market, or as citizens with rights under the law of the land? That these tensions have not been dealt with in the implementation of community care policy has left a grumbling uncertainty for the actors involved, all of whom, with the addition of front line workers, seem thrown together in a struggle for control, through the various means at their disposal, be it political action in the council chamber, or on the streets, management practice or discretionary practice by street level workers.

Managerialism may be the ideology behind this introduction, but what kind of management are we referring to? The requirements for management in this context are that it is controlling of vested interests and, therefore, that it is able to create transparent systems for the management (i.e. control) of the behaviour of key individuals. As James has pointed out this was 'not just any kind of management ... It came in industrial Tayloresque form' (James 1994; p.70). The Government did not want any uncertainties to creep into this 'revolution' as John Major referred to it when Chief Secretary to the Treasury, and the formulation therefore was classic scientific rational management theory involving characteristics which will be familiar to most people working in Social Services Departments:

- work determined by objectives which are specified both through task and targets
- task analysis leading to role specialisation
- activity grouped into 'functional units' (James 1994; p.46)
- line management to ensure clarity in both accountability and communication
- authority and responsibility delegated close to the task.

Efficiency, economy and effectiveness are the key objectives of this managerialist enterprise, although, as Pollitt has pointed out, there is evidence to suggest that the latter comes 'a poor third' as a priority (Pollitt 1993; p.138).   This has created 'task driven' (James 1994; p.47) organisations in which there was a 'separation of monitoring and control from the process of service delivery' (James 1994; p.48).   As James argues, this has enhanced rather than managed the tensions between control and professional practice that there used to be in welfare bureaucracies.   Separation, demarcation and 'keeping people ignorant' at the lower ends of organisations is what Argyris and Schon (1995) have used as part of their definition of the opposite of organisational learning. This pressure around the concept of professional discretion mirrors and helps to explain many of the stresses noted already in the first period of empirical research.   It will arise again when we return to the experience of care managers in chapter nine below.   'Resistance and inertia' (James 1994; p.49) in Social Services Departments for example could then be explained by the dominance of the classical model.   James is not the only author to equate explicitly or implicitly (Pollitt 1993) the introduction of scientific management with 'top down control' (James 1994; p.56) in policy implementation.   There is then, within Neo-Taylorist managerialism, a combination of decentralisation of authority and responsibility but within very strict systems of control - for example targets, contracting, financial control, staff appraisal, inspection, performance indicators, and information control.   The ideological imperative of 'marketisation' within managerialism creates a discourse of consumerism.   It is interesting and pertinent to note that consumerism creates and objectifies consumers as customers in managerialist terms. This plus the language of 'units of production' which are used to describe day care centres and residential homes, and 'packages of care' to describe sets of human relationships (Smale et al 1993) places this form of managerialism firmly within the positivist philosophy of scientific determinism, in much the same way that we will see social work knowledge doing within the medical model, in the next chapter.

James' (1994) argument on this subject concludes that such scientific managerialism is not suited to the flexibility required within (post) modern uncertainties.   She and other authors (Clarke, Cochrane and McLaughlin 1994; Williams 1994; Gerding 1993) speak of a 'new' managerialism as an alternative which we now turn to.

Strong claims have been made for contemporary concepts such as Total Quality Management (TQM) to represent a new paradigm in management theory (Morgan and Murgatroyd 1994). Unlike Taylorism, TQM does not offer a model for certainty, rather it assumes there are a network of relationships which create an organisational reality. The claims made for this 'paradigm wholeness' (Morgan and Murgatroyd 1994; p.x) are 'wholly subversive of many long-held assumptions.' (Morgan and Murgatroyd 1994; p.4) One of the key features which is of interest when making comparisons with traditional hierarchical forms of management is that the 'Total' refers partly to the intended involvement of the totality of the workforce. Quality of outcome is not the responsibility of senior managers and specialist quality control personnel alone, but of everyone within the organisation.

The language, within this new paradigm, is interesting in that it speaks of empowerment of the workforce. We shall note, in the next chapter, that contemporary social work literature is also full of empowerment as a form of discourse. What is the meaning of the term within TQM? The three statements 'managers are responsible' (Morgan and Murgatroyd 1994; p.5), 'workers at all levels must be empowered' to enhance all organisational processes (Morgan and Murgatroyd 1994; p.6) and 'only the customer can legitimately define ... what is quality' (Morgan and Murgatroyd 1994; p.7), indicate the confusion about who is being empowered within the model. This criticism is not based on clever selections of quotations from one text. As we shall see below, there are a number of problems with this new form of managerialism which are equally levelled at the more traditional approaches.

Mintzberg (1989) has also presented a differing model of management which offers the observation that 'any manager will quickly lay to rest the notion that managers practice a science' (Mintzberg 1989; p.14). Moving well away from the certainties of knowledge and technique which characterise Taylorist management theory, Mintzberg is keen to stress the importance of intuition, noting, for example, that 'managers' effectiveness is significantly influenced by their insight into their own work' (Mintzberg 1989; p.22). There are strong echoes within this thrust of the Mintzberg thesis of reflectiveness within social work practice (Schon 1987; Gould and Taylor 1996). He is not, however, speaking of unbridled and unreflective intuition, rather of seeking a balance between intuition and analysis. Factual analysis, for Mintzberg, needs to serve the purposes of service delivery and will be influenced not only by intuition and insight based upon experience, but also upon 'values'. He notes the problem of 'the rule of the tool' (Mintzberg 1989; p.56) and offers a powerful argument about failures to consider value in the face of hard facts. 'Facts become impregnated with value' (Mintzberg 1989; p64) so a 'basic moral reference point' (Mintzberg 1989; p64) is essential for analysis and decision-making. This, again, is very close to contemporary views of what social work should be about with the emphasis on 'value requirements' in the professional qualification (CCETSW 1995).

Mintzberg contrasts two forms of organisation which he argues are possibilities for the public sector. Firstly there are 'machine bureaucracies' obsessed with the pursuit of efficiency, a concept 'associated with criteria which are measurable' (Mintzberg 1989; p.332). This obsession with measurability is an example of a 'narrow form of rationality' (Mintzberg 1989; p.343) which 'drives out judgement and intuition' (Mintzberg 1989; p346). He contrasts this form of hierarchical, sanitized Taylorist organisation in which formal procedures rule human endeavour (Mintzberg 1989; p.351) rather than vice versa, with his ideal organisation which emphasises the importance of learning and the need to be constantly open to learning. Mintzberg's learning organisation is founded epistemologically on knowledge created through relationship, a form of rationality built upon intuitive rather than linear forms of reasoning (Mintzberg 1989; p.342). This is very close to the Argyris and Schon (1996) model described in chapter two, in which 'theory-in-use' is contrasted with an organisation's espoused theory. Although it may be largely tacit within an organisation, Argyris and Schon argue that theory-in-use, constructed within an organisation through mutual learning processes over time 'largely accounts for its identity' (Argyris and Schon 1996; p. 14). Organisationally such structures are non-hierarchical, representing networks built upon horizontal rather than vertical integration (Mintzberg 1989; p.370). In practice they are responsive to all constituents - workers, clients, citizens and owners (Mintzberg 1989; p.370) motivated more by consideration of the social benefits of outcome rather than economic benefits, even if the latter are more quantifiable.

Mintzberg has other supporters elsewhere for his vision of the learning organisation (Senge 1990; Tsang 1997; Beer 1985; Pottage and Evans 1994). The concept of systems as a theoretical basis to understanding the way in which organisations learn is a fundamental part of these approaches to learning organisations (Beer 1985; Senge 1990). Mutual learning within such networks is also definitive. Senge refers to 'learning how to learn together' (Senge 1990; p.3) at all levels within the organisation and he contrasts this approach with more traditional controlling organisations. Empowerment, for Senge, is, as with Mintzberg, a key to the effective learning organisation. All these authors note that the techniques of traditional authoritarian organisations tend to be 'prescriptive procedures' (Pottage and Evans 1994; p.12) that stifle creative development and, therefore, organisational learning. This analysis is very close to the concerns expressed in the earlier chapter (chapter four) in which the managerialism revealed in some of the key texts in care management was thought likely to be equally stifling of practice in such a complex area as assessment where flexibility and reflective use of discretion are important. Beer refers to the importance of 'requisite variety' (Beer 1985) to deal with such diversity and difference. A constructivist approach is also revealed in these authors' work. 'Through learning we re-create ourselves' declares Senge (Senge 1990; p. 14), whilst Pottage and Evans define learning organisations as those with 'policies based on the everyday meanings and understandings that are created by the interaction of workers and users' (Pottage and Evans 1994; p.16). Reflection and analysis of 'mental models' (Senge 1990; p. 9) is a key to the learning process and brings the concept of learning organisations close to contemporary approaches to social work theory (Gould and Taylor 1996). There is here a debt, perhaps, to Donald Schon's work on reflective learning for effective practice. Pottage and Evans' view of the competent workplace is built upon their work with a number of different social welfare agencies. The Schon thesis is compounded in their discovery, when engaged with these agencies, that 'skilful professional artistry' is more effective in dealing with the complexities of practice than practice broken down into measurable tasks, a managerial approach more in line with a traditional Taylorist model. We return to Schon and reflective practice in the next chapter.

Tsang (1997) adopts a more critical approach to the literature on learning organisations and organisational learning, noting that it is a contested concept in a range of literature, much of which is theoretically somewhat arid. He even questions the degree to which some conceptualisation of the term learning organisation requires there to be any identifiable cognitive or behavioural change, although the versions described above do more or less tacitly require there to be some change in understanding and behaviour within their definition of a competent or learning organisation. Tsang also usefully questions the nature of learning. Is it always such a good thing? Other writers are not always so critical of the nature of the learning in their rush to endorse the importance of learning within effective organisations. Tsang argues that static models of learning that are culturally specific, can have discriminatory consequences for those working within, or receiving services from, the organisation if their way of seeing or understanding is not validated by powerful ways of knowing and doing within the organisation.   Tsang then claims the importance of Kolb-like cycles of learning, moving through an iterative process in critical style towards good theory.   There is a congruence between these approaches to learning and that described later, in chapter eight, when a new conceptual framework for research practice is discussed. The model also helps in our search for a more helpful   conceptual framework to make sense of policy implementation, management and social work practice in the care management context.

There are other authors who have noted, through empirical work, the existence of these influences within the public sector (James 1994; Clarke, Cochrane and McLaughlin 1994; Williams 1994; Gerding 1993).   The key features of what is referred to as new management or new managerialism by these authors are much as described by Mintzberg.   The need for managers to 'create, maintain and continually improve' personal networks (Gerding op.cit.;p.185), provides the organisational description.   This is enhanced by continual delayering of hierarchies resulting in decentralisation in which control is maintained less through line management than the requirement to demonstrate the achievement of performance targets relating to an over all mission statement, and monitored through inspection techniques (Pollitt 1993; p.182).

Pollitt's observation of contemporary public sector organisation echoes the Morgan and Murgatroyd definition of TQM in which managers are 'allowed' to manage, but only within mission statements of objective set by senior managers.   Mintzberg is very wedded to the notion of innovation in learning organisations, generated by the freeing up of managers to use their intuitive and creative instincts, within organisational frameworks. Williams (1994; p.51) similarly describes 'a new managerialism able to initiate flexibility and respond quickly to new opportunities'.   This is, however, where the ideal type of TQM begins to unravel in practice, as it would seem that there is strong evidence that this freedom to act is limited to certain people within the organisation.   Rather than the Morgan and Murgatroyd model of 'Total' meaning everyone in the organisation, Williams notes that, in the post-Fordist interpretation, new managerialism has resulted in the de-skilling of many jobs (Williams 1994; p.54), and pointedly failed to pick up on the continuing tendency to 'universalise a white, male experience of work' (Williams 1994; p.56), thus failing to take account of the importance of difference and diversity which should be explicit within most concepts of empowerment (Braye and Preston-Shoot 1995).

There are other factors that need to be considered in this analysis of management theory which help us understand the managerial influence on policy implementation. Whilst there have been claims made for new management theory to be seen as a new paradigm (Morgan and Murgatroyd 1994), there is a counter argument that managerialism, whether old or new, still creates an overarching form of knowledge, or discourse as it was defined in chapter four. The ideology, as Clarke and his colleagues put it, insists on 'the commitment to management as the solution to social and economic problems ... the belief in management as an overarching system of authority, and the view of management as founded on an inalienable 'right to manage'' (Clarke et al 1994 ; p.16). This discourse of 'the right to manage' has become powerfully persuasive and, therefore, hard to challenge. Mintzberg, for instance, rather over-dramatically claims that 'no job is more vital to our society than that of the manager.' (Mintzberg 1989; p.24).

Other writers have questioned this right to manage by exploring accountability and legitimacy more generally, noting that the right to manage conflicts with other rights which hold some legitimacy, such as the rights of citizens and consumers (Taylor et al 1992). The legitimation of management has come about through political discourse, backed up by the actions of organisations such as the Audit Commission rather than through participatory or representative forms of democracy. Indeed, it could be argued that the introduction of management into the public sphere, inspired by the previous Conservative Government, was partly an attempt to undermine local democracy.

This brings us into the next area of critique in which the concepts of need and rights are contrasted. The language of TQM, it will be remembered, speaks of the supremacy of the consumer and yet places the responsibility for the creation of the mission statement - the statement of objectives - in the hands of senior management. This equates closely to the separation that has occurred in Social Services Departments, for example, in which the rhetoric of service user needs being paramount has been undermined by the requirement on Social Services Departments to be the prime movers in defining what the needs are that the Department will meet. It is managers then that define needs (Clarke et al 1994; p.6) In this sense, even within new managerialism, management remains exclusive rather than inclusive, controlling rather than empowering, and unencumbered by the requirements of political accountability and legitimation that are imposed on other actors in the implementation process. As Pollitt has noted (Pollitt 1993; p.187) new management is 'not so much a charter for citizen empowerment as managerialism with a human face'.

There is another conceptual arena - that of morality and values - in which we can criticise managerialism as a unified form of knowledge rather than two distinct paradigms - old and new. Bamford (Bamford 1989) notes four ways in which managerialism undermines concepts of morality. Interestingly he makes no distinction between new managerialist organisations and old bureaucracies, thus posing the question, what, with all the organisational change that has taken place, has actually shifted as far as the ethical underpinning of service delivery is concerned? Social relations in organisations such as Social Services Departments are defined impersonally.   There are powerful mechanisms which stereotype and categorise service users. We can now see these as the discursive practices of eligibility criteria and other forms of prioritisation or targeting.   The second way in which there is a degree of moral undermining is through increasing specialisation. This not only undermines the non-specialists - usually the care-givers - but also results, as does the process of categorisation, in the distancing of workers from 'ordinary moral responses' (Bamford 1989; p. 148).   Formal rules and procedures for decision-making, within the context of agency mission statements, have the effect of reinforcing 'the sense of distance between worker and client' (Bamford 1989; p.148).   Finally Bamford argues that personal obligation in the worker/client relationship is 'subordinated to organisational requirements' (Bamford 1989; p.148).   The Kantian ethic, so powerful within social work values (Jordan 1990; Banks 1995; Wilmot 1997), is then undermined by the utilitarianism of agency rules and regulations. This clash between managerialist values and social work values leads us into the next chapter where we will look more closely at social work knowledge, including values.

There is, however, a broader sense in which there is a clash between managerialism and more traditional forms of organisation for the distribution of social welfare. This concerns the undermining of the public service ethos by the introduction of a market in welfare services and the commodification of service users, principally through the introduction of managerialism and managerialist organisation. Peters (Peters 1993) notes the way that privatisation 'threatens some of the most fundamental values of the public sector' (Peters 1993; p.56). Replacing the 'values of public service with those of the market' has resulted in the substitution of 'one narrow conception of efficiency for more fundamental values of accountability and responsiveness' (Peters 1993; p.56). Flynn (1990) has characterised this split between the new right approach to the sector and the public service ethic as individualism, private ownership, profit and market forces arrayed against collective responsibility, equitable treatment and the belief that making profits from essential services is morally wrong. Flynn describes the future of public sector as a battle for control by these two sets of values. 'Whose values predominate depends on who is most powerful' (Flynn 1990; p.172).

In a somewhat rhetorical and certainly impassioned argument, Stewart and Ransom argue the requirement of a 'publicly established concept of need' (Stewart and Ransom 1988; p.56). They introduce concepts of equity and justice into the debate, much as Mintzberg would, claiming that 'it is not sufficient to ask whether management is efficient, it must also be asked whether it is just' (Stewart and Ransom 1988; p.58). Their argument is for the fundamental right of clients of public service organisations to be seen as citizens with rights equal to those of the people who manage and deliver the service. As we have seen above, the ability to define need becomes the more powerful discursive opportunity than the rights of individuals. As Potter argues in the same volume (Potter 1988), consumerism only addresses one form of relationship - that between the consumer and the market. There is no concept of the collective as there is in more rights based approaches to citizenship. 'Perhaps', Potter argued perceptively, as long ago as 1988, 'this explains why consumerist principles stop at representation instead of moving on to embrace participation' (Potter 1998 p.257). With consumerism there is only the option of 'exit' from the market place - perhaps best defined as Hobson's choice for the vast majority of marginalised service users who do not have access to private health and social care. With citizenship and participation there is the opportunity for *voice*. Managerialism, however, has fundamental problems in hearing voice. Within managerialist discourse, as Carter and Jackson argue, the voice of the consumer is no more than 'the voice of the object of motivational strategies, whose role is simply to be passively manipulated' (Carter and Jackson 1993; p.95).

What, finally, happens when you put managerialism, whether it be of the new or the old variety, into the world of finite resources' (Flynn 1990)? Once people who are potential users of welfare services have had their expectations raised by talk of their needs being met, whether it be within a context of consumerism or a broader version of citizenship and rights, who makes the decisions about priorities? There is no facility to commission more hours of domiciliary service, like more hours of television piped or beamed into our homes when the demand increases, because, unlike the potential market for television viewing, there are strict limits on expenditure which are at the mercy of the Public Sector Borrowing Requirement. 'Competitive mechanisms', driven by a managerialist agenda, then have 'at least as much to do with driving down unit costs as with promoting quality' (Pollitt 1993). With a clear echo of Mintzberg's ethical approach, Stewart and Ransom (Stewart and Ransom 1994; p.66) urge that 'the management of rationing requires an understanding and an assessment of need' which is not necessary in the private sector. Professional and political judgements about entitlement are not the same as judgements about marketability (Flynn 1990; p. 180) so, as Flynn goes on to argue, there are major problems in 'the wholesale importation of private sector management techniques and the ideologies that go with them' (Flynn 1990; p.180/1) into a welfare quasi-market. The language of managerialist resource control, built upon the   reality of resource constraint, is a recipe for conflict with a professional workforce that has claims to be motivated by a public service ethic in which the concept of relationship is deeper than 'have a nice day!' (Flynn 1990; p.144).

So what does social work, mediated through the practice of care managers, have as an alternative body of knowledge to contrast with the managerialist set of values? There is, as has been indicated above, a deep feeling amongst care managers and first line managers (chapter three) that managerialism is a marginalising force for social work values. The end of discretion, I have argued, is a premature forecast. We have noted, within the learning organisations debate, that there is the beginnings of a new approach to organisational culture that is at odds with new and old forms of managerialism. So how might care managers who are social workers use their professional knowledge to inform that discretion?

7 Care Management and Social Work Theory

Introduction

The main research questions for this book require the exploration of the limits to policy implementation, and, within the illustrative example, examination of the extent to which key implementers such as care managers might undermine the intentions of community care policy makers by the use of ill-considered discretion. In this chapter the focus moves to social work and the theoretical knowledge that social workers have at their disposal to inform their practice. In order to contain the discussion about social work knowledge, the focus will be on assessment practice, as was the case with the fieldwork carried out with care managers, described in chapter three. Assessment is, as we have noted, a key activity in care management (SSI 1991a; SSI 1991b). Although many practitioners have an assessment role in community care, both qualified and pre-qualified, it is still social workers who are most likely to be carrying out assessments, so it is the potential knowledge base for social work practice which will be analysed in this chapter.

The task at this stage is that I should address the opportunities within the knowledge base available to social workers for informing a professional practice which fits in with the approaches to policy implementation that I have described in this book.

To what extent, then, does theory for social work provide validation for the concept that assessment is about the management of scarce resources on the one hand or about the exploration of need through the construction of meaning and identity on the other? I noted in chapter three that there was evidence in the interviews of two different forms of professionalism. The first, traditional, approach, is based upon a positivist interpretation of expertise which assumes social workers will accumulate knowledge that they then utilise in making judgements about other people's needs. The second approach, the more contemporary version of professionalism, recognises that need is a relative term that requires exploration of meaning and that the best method of approaching this is through a participatory approach to assessment practice. The more contemporary approach is also informed by the argument put forward by Doyal and Gough (1991) who claim that the fundamental requirement in decision-making for individuals before their 'intermediate needs' can be met (Doyal and Gough 1991) is that of autonomy. A traditional expert approach to professionalism can be placed in contrast to more contemporary versions that seek to empower service users and enhance their opportunities for autonomy and decision-making.

In addition, chapter three also noted that there was a bureaucratic application of practice techniques in which managerialist systems were put into effect largely outside of either of these professional models for practice. Such an approach as this would match with the rationalist expectations for 'perfect implementation' which has been seen as so problematic.

Where can we find, within social work theory, evidence of a knowledge base that indicates the traditional perspective on professionalism? Which social work theory is more in tune with the managerial agenda of rationalist policy implementation? Or, conversely, where might social workers look for a knowledge base that enables them to adopt a participative and empowering practice in relation to potential service users who are often marginalised and have great difficulties, as a result of perhaps mental health problems, such as dementia, or learning difficulties, in having their voice heard and their needs met?

There is a strong belief that the practice of social work within care management has been marginalised by a shift to a more budget-led and bureaucratised agenda for social work affected by the broader influences of privatization and globalization (Dominelli and Hoogvelt 1996). In this chapter, however, I will not look at the bureaucratic and organisational construction of assessment in social services departments, but rather dwell on the knowledge and skills which practitioners might be drawing upon to inform their practice, when instrumentation gives them some leeway to express professional discretion as it was seen to do in chapter three. To attempt such an enterprise is to open a window on a long standing debate in social work education and research about the link between theory and action in social work practice (Curnock and Hardiker 1979; Hardiker and Barker 1981). In setting the scene it is important to acknowledge this debate and the complexity, in practice, of the relationship between what is written and what is done. Consequently the chapter needs to analyse critically theoretical knowledge for social work, and it does so in a number of ways. There is reference to Rojek's (1986) concept of the 'gladiatorial paradigm' which criticises the battle for supremacy in meaning in social work knowledge as a false expectation. As will be seen, the participative approach to social work practice argued in this chapter deconstructs this gladiatorial paradigm. The body of knowledge usually referred to as 'values' or ethics for social work (Jordan 1990; Banks 1995; Hugman and Smith 1995; Wilmot 1997) also provides an interesting critique of objectivism in the traditional perspective on professional expertise. The central importance of voice in the contemporary value base to social work practice provides a convincing deconstruction of traditional ownership of expertise in professional practice because of the way in which it acknowledges that service users can be experts in their own circumstances and that the process of assessment is one of a collaborative exploration of those needs between the service user and the enabling worker. Lastly there is some discussion of the concept of reflection (Schon 1987; Gould and Taylor 1996) which provides an explanation of the process by which theory and practice are merged. This critical process provides opportunities for social workers to seek clarity about the nature of the knowledge base they are utilising as they strive to develop effectiveness in their practice.

It was first observed in chapter three that there is evidence of both traditional and more contemporary social work discourse in the practice of care managers. As I have argued, traditional professionalism assumes an expertise on the part of the practitioner which enables them to apply techniques to particular circumstances which will ensure a successful outcome (Schon 1987). This level of scientific rationality is contrasted with an approach which views practice as a process of exploration, of making sense of social reality, often across cultural divides. The claims to this kind of paradigm separation mirror very much that noted above between traditional management theory and approaches such as TQM (Morgan and Murgatroyd 1994) in the previous chapter. Having acknowledged the problem of scientific rationality in its attempts to pin down the reality of human behaviour, it is important to explore the extent to which social work theory reflects the modernist enterprise of scientific rationalism or whether there are, within social work theory, forms of knowledge that offer social workers opportunities to draw upon knowledge in a more critical and reflective manner (Parton 1994; Howe 1994). I will, therefore, be analysing some of the different forms of knowledge available to see how social work theory reflects social constructivist or positivist world views.

In as much as the care managers interviewed in the first set of empirical work were apparently engaged in unreflective use of discretion which was undermining of policy intentions, it is important that this chapter facilitates some understanding of the degree to which social work theory lends support to unbridled use of discretion or enables the use of a more critical and reflective approach. Such deliberations will cast useful light upon the extent to which policy intentions are *inevitably* undermined by implementers such as care managers in the way that Lipsky has described Street Level Bureaucrats behaviour (Lipsky 1980). The alternative is that social workers might engage either individually or collectively in constructing practice around policy guidelines through a process of reflection and in a condition of participation and collaboration with all stakeholders - politicians, managers, colleagues and service users. This may allow for a more deliberately creative use of discretion in the pursuit of policy implementation.

There have been a number of attempts to categorise theoretical perspectives on social work practice (Whittington and Holland 1985; Howe 1987; Payne 1991). These commentaries at least imply that there are traditional, managerialist and more contemporary approaches to social work revealed within these theories, but it is important to acknowledge here, the dangers of adopting what has been termed a 'gladiatorial paradigm' (Rojek 1986; p. 66), in which opposing epistemologies compete for the right to define essential reality. Rojek has criticised what he refers to as 'subject centred theories' (Rojek 1986; p. 69) in which social work is characterised as something that is done to clients (sic) identified as subjects within social work practice. Rojek argues from a post-structuralist approach to social work practice, which he claims would avoid the dangers of this spurious battle for meaning and tendency for theory to construct subjects. My argument is that a participative approach deconstructs the gladiatorial paradigm and enables social workers to work with colleagues, service users and others to construct a real world that has mutual meaning, or at the least mutual understanding.

Social Work Theory and Rationalism

To what extent, then, do different forms of social work theory reflect the scientific rationalism that we have seen at play within policy implementation and managerialist theory in previous chapters? Within psycho-dynamic casework (Hamilton 1951; Hollis 1972), the word assessment is displaced by the term diagnosis in the literature, placing it within a medical model. Diagnosis analyses the problems of an individual's functioning through the application of a theory of personality structure. Overcoming personal difficulties through treatment follows a successful diagnosis of the manner in which there is a disparity between the individual and a developmental norm.

Despite the criticisms of psycho-dynamic diagnosis as a method of assessment, the influence on current social work practice remains considerable (Payne 1991). Criticisms of psycho-dynamic theory have been on a number of grounds, including effectiveness and a failure to stand up to empirical testing (Sheldon 1986), the binding of the practice to an illusory structural concept (e.g. Krill in Payne 1991), and the failure to take into account the extent to which a dominant social structure might oppress some groups (Ahmad 1991; Corrigan and Leonard 1978). It has also been argued that psycho-dynamic casework employs 'quasi-medical approaches that regard people as subjects for treatment' (Adams 1996; p.19). Psycho-dynamic casework, is, in this argument, built upon a knowledge construct that objectifies individuals in much the same way as managerialism was shown to in the previous chapter. These criticisms have not succeeded in undermining the influence of the approach. Whilst it would seem that psycho-dynamic casework fits within the scientific rationalist model, to conclude as much denies the hermeneutic way in which the theory is often used in social work practice.

Social workers using a behaviourist approach adopt a role of change agent, demonstrating 'an ability to analyse people's behaviour ... the nature ... of their interactions ... the ability to form testable hypotheses ... and a repertoire of effective intervention methods' (Hudson and Macdonald 1986). Assessment in this model is about identifying problem behaviour, its context, its antecedents and its consequences.

The effectiveness of different approaches is clearly of great importance to political (D of H 1989) and managerial (Challis and Davies 1986) influences on community care practice. There is evidence to concur that behaviourism is the method to pursue if effectiveness is the goal (Sheldon 1986). Behavioural social work is an excellent method for identifying problems, categorising them according to agency priorities and instituting quick and (at least superficially) effective intervention before passing on to the next person battering at the door. Behaviourism, within social work theory, as within psychology, is the scientific rationalist approach par excellence. It provides the social worker with the expert knowledge and the techniques of application to go with it. It offers the positivist benefits of predictability and replicability, as evidence from Sheldon's research into effectiveness demonstrates (Sheldon 1986). The positivist failing of dealing only with problem formulations that can most easily be defined (Thompson 1995), together with an underlying ethos of control, however, puts behaviourism outside of the more empowering approaches of modern social work discourse.

Family therapy theory is another area of influence on social work (Barker 1986). The structure of 'diagnostic formulation' is familiar - description of problem, family constitution, therapist's understanding of family problems and their maintenance, strengths and motivation to change, and 'ecological context or supra-system' (Barker 1986). Following this process, feedback is offered to the family. As with other theoretical perspectives which employ a medical model, this approach to family therapy involves professional judgement. The lack of service user participation in assessment suggests that systemic family therapy has little to offer social work practice in assessment as informed by contemporary professional and political agendas that emphasise a participative approach and a service user focus.

'Assessment', says Epstein in her handbook on the Task Centred Approach (Epstein 1980), 'consists of finding out the problems (exploration), together with classification and specification of the problem.' Despite this use of the word exploration, task centred casework is a tool to be drawn upon by those motivated by a managerial agenda. The most influential writers on care management from the managerial tendency (Challis and Davies 1986) cite the task centred approach as most nearly matching care management as they propose it (Challis and Davies 1986; p.45).

Task centred practice is described as both a 'technology' (Reid and Epstein 1972), and a 'set of procedures' (Epstein 1980). Assessment is described as the process that 'places a person in some service classification' (Epstein 1980). A model of assessment that so clearly links targeted needs to available services, is very attractive to those with an eye on efficiency and cost effectiveness and is at odds with needs-led approaches. From the point of view of outcome effectiveness the task centred approach has a good record (Reid and Epstein 1972; Goldberg et al 1984). Day (1993) cites the influence of organisational factors revealed in the Goldberg research. He adds that 'the model is attractive to social service managers seeking clearly defined goals for services which are achievable and where costs as well as outcomes can be clearly monitored' (Day 1993). This attractiveness raises substantial concerns about how realistic is the wish that 'the target problem is what a client thinks is the problem' (Epstein 1980). Research quoted by Day (Day 1993) from the Doel and Marsh book on the subject (Doel and Marsh 1993) suggests that failure to agree goals is likely to reduce effectiveness. Task centred casework can only sustain its effectiveness within a perspective of empowerment, although assessment is seen as 'a judgement of use to practitioners. It seems to be of little direct use to clients' (Epstein 1980; p 219).

Assessment, in the model, is a move beyond the targeting of priority problems, and is concerned with defining those problems. This process of definition provides clear echoes of a behaviourist approach - when and how often does the target problem occur? with whom and where? with what antecedents and what consequences? (Epstein 1980 p 219). To suggest that the definition of a target problem is of no concern to service users takes the Epstein version well beyond contemporary social work interests, as well as the rhetoric of the political agenda for community care. This leaves the model more in the hands of managerialism as managers fulfil their responsibilities, defining needs and managing them within scarce resources.

It would be possible to use a task centred approach in an empowering and needs-led fashion (Doel and Marsh 1992). The model for the practice of assessment, however, with its emphasis on the definition of limited priority targets, an expectation of short term intervention, employing methodologies that are of proven effectiveness, and with more than a wink towards behaviourism, makes the method more a tool for the rationing of scarce resources, and brings it firmly within a rationalist perspective for managerialism and policy implementation.

Crisis Intervention is another model for practice with some relevance within the practice sphere, as managers in social services departments draft community care plans which include areas of priority that the agency is committed to dealing with. This is the discursive practice of community care that places the responsibility for needs and priority definition in the hands of management in social services departments. The degree to which these needs are determined as a result of real collaboration with service users has not been adequately tested as yet. Care managers, as we have noted in chapter three are concerned at the way in which priority matrices and eligibility criteria define those in greatest need as being individuals whose informal networks of support have failed. This system requires practitioners effectively to wait until a crisis occurs before they are allowed to intervene and provide a service. Crisis intervention, as a social work theory and practice, only deals with the assessment and resolution of crisis situations. As these are currently the prime focus for eligibility within care management assessment criteria, crisis intervention would seem to be an attractive proposition.

In its traditional (Parad 1968) and revised (O'Hagan 1986) forms, the scope of the theory is very limited - the individual or the family. Other criticisms involve a failure to take into account structural pressures such as racism, homophobia, heterosexism, disability and sexism. The focus, in Thompson's re-visitation of crisis intervention (Thompson 1991), is on assessing strengths as well as difficulties, looking to resources as well as noting the difficulties of those concerned to develop problem-solving skills. Assessment of the potential for harnessing resources within the community is seen as important. This focus on positive resources puts Thompson's model within the remit of current professional concerns with empowerment of service users, which is also a concern of the political agenda. Whilst crisis intervention does serve these influences to some degree, however, there is no doubt that the greatest appeal will be to managers who are keen to focus primarily on potential service users with the highest priority. Crisis intervention offers the illusion of a theoretical model that enables managers to urge practitioners to target those in greatest need - a rationalist expectation.

Social Work Theory and Participation in the Construction of Meaning

What forms of knowledge for social work are there which might counter those analysed above which adopt the largely scientific rationalist approach sometimes referred to within care management practice with older and disabled people as the medical model (Oliver 1996)? Humanism as an influence forms the second strand to Payne's paradigm for social work (Payne 1991). Interestingly enough, Rogers (1951), an influential writer about humanist counselling, is not interested in assessment or diagnosis. His starting point is the uniqueness of the individual and the importance of self-actualisation. Humanism's influence has been more upon the value base of social work than as a model for practice, although

England (1986) describes the process of a 'constant set of approximations' in the search for meaning between worker and client. 'Making sense' of the client's real world is a fundamental part of the process of harnessing the individual's strengths in coping, and thus overcoming their particular difficulty. The humanist ethos in practice seeks to avoid classification of individuals whose unique wholeness is respected. As a result, there is little likelihood of intervention being contaminated by the needs of resource rationing. Indeed, the lack of clear targets is one of the major criticisms of humanist intervention. Where these approaches achieve greatest congruence with current influence on assessment practice is in the way that they value differing realities - different cultural perspectives. Writers with a black perspective have for many years (Ahmed 1978 in Dominelli 1988; Gilroy 1987) criticised the way in which services are designed from an ethnocentric position. Such assessments are likely to discount people whose view of their own needs do not equate with service delivery criteria. A humanist ethic, with an existentialist view of reality might be a powerful starting point for an empowering, user-led, practice. On the other hand, for social workers operating within a context of resource management, such an ethic might well prove to be the blue touch paper that ignites burn out.

Community profiling is another form of assessment which, in its contemporary formulation adopts a user-led and empowering rationale that assumes the collective views of the community in question, democratically expressed, form the basis of assessment (Hawtin 1994). Indeed, there are many features of the practice of community profiling which reveal considerable congruence with both the political rhetoric of community care, and contemporary professional social work notions of good practice. The emphasis upon the expressed needs of local people is a fundamental strand of needs-led assessment, and makes this an important part of the process of an agency addressing the service user agenda. Services require planning on both an individual and authority-wide basis according to these expressed needs.

In this context it is important to notice the congruence between community profiling as both form of knowledge and technique with contemporary views of social work as empowerment (see below) and empowerment approaches to management. Community profiling is removed from the positivism of scientific rationalism by the ethos of user-centredness and the centrality of the concept of voice. It is not a case of the professional application of techniques to a given problem in order to establish a measurable outcome but rather a process of exploration which values the expressed views of the subjects who construct the community of interest. There is also congruence with participative research methodology which will be explored in the next chapter.

Anti-oppressive practice has developed as a concept, with growing theoretical base, in the wake of the perceived failure by many other theoretical perspectives to address the nature of oppression experienced by the majority of social welfare service users, and the consequent inability to develop a practice which seeks to empower people rather than replicate the oppression they experience. It is, therefore, an approach that is allied closely to that of TQM and empowerment approaches in managerialism, at least according to the claims of TQM protagonists (Morgan and Murgatroyd 1994). Empowerment in social work is epistemologically separate from the positivism of the medical and scientific rationalist approaches covered above, in as much as it seeks to give voice to those who are most likely to be users of social and welfare services, and whose general experience will have been one of marginalisation and oppression. Humanism is the only theoretical concept that adopts a constructivist approach to human relationships in an ontological sense.

Anti-oppressive practice has been developed almost exclusively as a result of the struggles of oppressed people - most notably black people, disabled people, women and gay men and women. In his critique of family therapy, Howe suggests the need to develop a practice based less on 'scientifically styled therapeutic technique' (Howe 1989; p89), than 'one which takes the individual's experience as the basis of social theorising' (Howe 1989; p.113). It is the latter that defines anti-oppressive and empowering approaches.

The other theoretical base to empowerment and anti-oppression is power. The discursive practices that construct community care (chapter four) are forms of power that implicitly or explicitly fail to 'amend the ideology of white superiority that is an essential feature of racism' (Braye and Preston-Shoot 1995; p.101). The same process occurs in disability, patriarchy, ageism, mental health and heterosexism, in which dominant forms of knowledge and therefore action, determine the context in which services are provided and marginalise those whose experience does not match the dominant ideology. Anti-oppressive social work is built upon this understanding and requires practitioners to deconstruct power relationships which social workers have traditionally upheld, and work in closer partnership (Braye and Preston-Shoot 1995) with service users and local communities to enable people to define their own reality.

Basing theory on the direct experience of disadvantaged people results in a practice which is informed by an understanding of power relationships (Gould 1992; Dalrymple and Burke 1995). As well as involving practice which is intended to enable people to take back control over the decisions that affect their lives, anti-oppressive practice also means the honest and open acknowledgement of power differentials when they occur, for example in decision-making for service provision (Baldwin 1996b). The stress on user definition of need and empowering people to take control over their own welfare, again puts this practice at the centre of contemporary wisdom on good social work practice, allying it with the rhetoric of political influence on community care, and making a start at addressing the service user agenda.

The literature on empowerment not only describes a practice for assessment (Ahmad 1990; p26; Dalrymple and Burke 1995, p.114; Braye and Preston-Shoot; Hughes 1995), but also provides a useful critique for the practice of assessment using both agency instrumentation and other theoretical perspectives on social work practice. Ahmad's (Ahmad 1990) critique of task-centred and unitary approaches to social work are examples. Research (Ellis 1993; Baldwin 1995) has suggested that agency instrumentation is service-led, does not promote user or carer participation, and needs to be determined by an understanding of disadvantage as well as other factors. Research has also demonstrated how theoretical models such as the medical model of disability still informs much practice in community care assessments (Ellis 1993). This was the case in my interpretation of the knowledge base for practice revealed in many of the interviews with care managers described in chapter three above. Care managers were not only adopting a medical model, but also a traditional professionalism that regarded assessment as a professional opinion, based on previously acquired knowledge, not as a result of a process of participation which is more the intentions of contemporary user-led and anti-oppressive approaches.

The theory of anti-oppressive practice is, therefore, one that can usefully inform the exploratory influence on social work assessment. Where priorities have to be made between competing demands, and services have to be rationed, empowerment approaches ensure that all competing demands should be considered. The practice of distributing welfare resources is then based on principles of equity rather than greatest need as defined by management within organisations that are still largely oppressive (Braye and Preston-Shoot 1995). We have already heard from practitioners (chapter three) that targeting those most in need is an ineffective method of distributing scarce resources. It results in organisations waiting until informal networks of support break down before services are provided. This is a far from equitable basis for distribution and would clearly discriminate against individuals, families or communities who already feel marginalised from mainstream service provision. Anti-oppressive practice should ensure that the most vulnerable and least powerful groups should get the greatest access to decision-making processes. Empowerment in social work, in as much as it is at odds with the certainties of scientific rationalism, provides a useful brake on the more objectivist approaches to rationing in social services departments. There are convincing claims (Adams 1996) that the move in social work practice from 'client treatment to citizen empowerment' (Adams 1996; p.20) is a paradigm shift, in much the same way that Murgatroyd and Morgan (1994) claim TQM is such a paradigm shift.

Making a claim for anti-discriminatory and anti-racist practice in the way described above is a potentially dangerous game. To put these expectations of empowerment alongside the arguments in previous chapters of systematic undermining of policy intentions (for good or ill) and the tales of self-protective behaviour detailed by Lipsky (1980) and Satyamurti (1981), might suggest that the contemporary knowledge base for social work practice is hopelessly idealistic. How might such a criticism be analysed? There is a claim made later in this chapter that there is a well-argued methodology for a social work practice in care management which addresses the combination of the exploration of human needs within the resource constraint imperative (Smale et al 1993). In this later section these concerns will be looked at in some detail.

Values in Social Work Practice

CCETSW (1995) regulations stipulate that students pursuing the Diploma in Social Work must demonstrate the 'value requirements' through the 'core competences' that define the curriculum for practice placements. These values require students to:

- 'identify and question their own values and prejudices, and their implications for practice;
- respect and value uniqueness and diversity, and recognise and build on strengths;

- promote people's right to choice, privacy, confidentiality and protection, while recognising and addressing the complexities of competing rights and demands;
- assist people to increase control of and improve the quality of their lives, while recognising that control of behaviour will be required at times in order to protect children and adults from harm;
- identify, analyse and take action to counter discrimination, racism, disadvantage, inequality and injustice, using strategies appropriate to role and function;
- practise in a manner that does not stigmatise or disadvantage either individuals, groups or communities' (CCETSW 1995).

Despite the problems that care managers had in articulating the values that underpinned their practice when asked in the fieldwork interviews analysed above, it is strongly argued that it is 'impossible to have value-free knowledge' (Banks 1995; p.66). All of the theoretical perspectives defined in this chapter hold, implicitly or explicitly, a system of values within them. If the CCETSW requirements provide the definitive contemporary version then it is interesting to note which of the theories above are fully inclusive. This test is unfair in the sense that values are not absolute and outside of social or historical conditions and many of those listed above have been articulated only fairly recently within mainstream social work knowledge.

It is now widely believed that the open articulation of values through reflective practice is the best and perhaps only way of ensuring that oppressive practices that subvert the intentions of social work are not present when social workers engage with service users (Baldwin 1996b; Banks 1995; Jordan 1990; Hugman and Smith 1995; Wilmot 1997). On this rating it can be argued that there are problems with much of the knowledge revealed above. Most of the theoretical perspectives and practice models are built upon a traditional, individual and pathological approach. They fall within the medical model which is largely problem focused, so will tend not to 'recognise and build upon strengths'. (CCETSW 1995) In addition the more traditional approach to the use of professional knowledge means that the use of models such as behaviourism, task-centred social work or crisis intervention, are going to be less easy to use in promoting people's rights to choice, and in assisting them to increase control of their lives. The individual focus may well be geared towards the traditional approach of social services departments to assessment and care planning, but it does not encompass the community orientation to need implied in much of the community care policy literature, especially relating to participation with local communities to establish their view of collective needs.   This sort of paradigm clash compounds the problems of confusion and incongruence in community care discourse revealed in chapter four.

The values expressed in the CCETSW document are most closely associated with anti-oppressive and empowerment approaches to social work practice, located within a humanist perspective. This, with the more contemporary requirement to address provision of services within resource constraints, makes the matching of social work knowledge - both practice theory and values - with agency requirements, a hard task to fulfil. We now look at one model for practice that attempts to blend together these forms of knowledge into a coherent form of knowledge to support contemporary social work practice, including that within the care management arena.

The Exchange Model - a More Useful Epistemology for Care Management Practice?

Smale and his colleagues (Smale et al 1993) moot three approaches to social work practice. The Exchange model is one of these. The other two are the Questioning and the Procedural approaches.   The Questioning model involves practitioners using professional expertise to make sense of potential service users' needs and then prescribe packages of services which would best meet those needs. The Questioning model is the traditional professional approach which was used by some care managers as was seen from some of the evidence available within the interviews in chapter three.

The Procedural model is bureaucratic in essence and assumes that managers will demonstrate their 'expertise in setting criteria for resource allocation' (Smale et al 1993). This, we can see, equates very closely to the managerial agenda that has been argued as the dominant influence on current practice, even if it is strongly resisted by many practitioners.   The Procedural approach, espousing efficiency and cost effectiveness, and propounding, as it does, strictly organisational responses to need, involves ideas that, in the eighties and nineties, found their time in history. Senior managers, embracing the residual political ideology of market influence on the provision of welfare services, are still influential in social services departments. To allow welfare provision for vulnerable citizens to become subject to the vagaries of the market when the government is struggling with budget deficit places services and those who depend on them at great risk.

Social work practice, as informed by the theoretical perspectives outlined above, is under pressure from the same quarters. This can happen because of lack of clarity in the theoretical position of social workers, or because of uncritical adherence to particular epistemological perspectives. We have evidence of a lack of clarity from the first fieldwork interviews. The apparent lack of reflectiveness in or upon practice by these practitioners leaves them open to being buffeted by managerial considerations, although they maintain some opportunities for the use of ill-considered discretion as Street Level Bureaucrats.

Lastly, many of the theoretical models that social workers draw upon are firmly within the scientific rationalist discourse, defined as part of the modernist project (Parton 1994; Howe 1994). Even though these two authors write persuasively of the fragmentation of the certainties that social work theory and practice have been built upon in its brief history, it is less easy for a critical theory, let alone a critical practice to develop within social work. If assessment is a key task for care management, so it is a fundamental part of social work, as we have seen above, in either its technical, medical (diagnostic) model, or within a more contemporary user-led and participatory mode. 'Classification', then, as a professional activity, is 'at the heart of social work discourse' (Rojeck et al 1988; p.137). The problem for social work theory and practice in rationalist exposition is that attempts to capture the reality of an individual's needs through technical or scientific means are being challenged by the concept of voice. Feminist, black, disabled, and, increasingly, gay and lesbian perspectives now challenge 'the assumption that particular theories might be capable of explaining the experiences of all clients' (Howe 1994). Social workers, as care managers, then have the choice either to behave as traditional professionals, classifying and defining service users, through their power in deciding 'what knowledge is to count as relevant' (Howe 1994; p.525/6), or to adopt a participatory approach in which they share that power to define, or even hand it over to service users to establish their own definition of what their needs are. It has been noted elsewhere in this book that the phrase 'needs-led' which had such an empowering ring to it at its inception has now been seriously deconstructed by the more contemporary phrase 'user-led'. Needs are, through the legislation

(HMSO 1990), defined by local authorities and interpreted through the discretionary practices of care managers. Care managers have a fundamental choice whether to use this opportunity to wield power or to share it. This is a question of behaviour, but it is also an issue of epistemology. What forms of knowledge will care managers draw upon to inform their practice when working with marginalised service users? We have noted the way in which traditional practice has been largely built upon the certainties of psychologically and medically based expert knowledge. Are care managers now allowing a new age of certainty built upon technocratic procedures to dominate their practice or is there a theoretical model, with a supportive value base and approach to practice that might combat such marginalising and discriminatory practices?

The conclusion we are moving towards is a pessimistic one. Despite the best intentions of any theoretical model in practice, the reality is that there are influences so powerful that the practice of such theories is either squeezed in line with dominant ideology, or it is pushed aside. So does social work theory and practice, shrug and accept its role as 'local government function' rather than profession (Bamford 1989), or do social workers hold on to the shreds of an ideological tradition that has developed? How real is the paradigm shift that Adams (Adams 1996) espouses in the sense that it could, as a form of knowledge, challenge more dominant ways of knowing and practising? Resources are scarce, but should we accept this as the motivating factor for decision-making in welfare agencies? Is there a different ideology that rejects the amorality of the market and argues that the best way to offer choice and hear voice is to recognise the way control - in defining needs and how best to meet them - has been denied to service users, and determines a practice aimed at sharing or handing back the power and opportunities to determine life chances?

There are two reasons why social work should retain a central place in the practice of assessment in community care. One is that social work ideology, in the contemporary professional light in which this chapter has cast it, largely converges with the political rhetoric of community care policy, and reflects the spirit of the community care legislation (HMSO 1990). Both at least claim to be interested in the service user agenda (voice and choice). The second reason borrows from the managerial agenda. In order for service delivery to be effective, that is to meet the aims originally intended, and for it to do this efficiently, resources must not be wasted by mis-application. For a needs-led assessment to have any chance of fruitful outcome, there must be at the least some theoretical relationship between what is assessed, and what is or might be available to meet those needs. Someone must know, firstly what is feasible, and secondly what the likely outcome is of a person using that service over a period of time. Does day care relieve the stress of loneliness? Does it always do this? Under what circumstances might this not be the outcome?

This is an issue of quality, and quality is a product of evaluation. If community care is about choice and standards, as the White Paper indicates (D of H 1989), then practice, including the provision of services, needs to be *evaluated*. In order for it to be evaluated effectively practitioners need to adopt a theoretical stance that takes us beyond implicit practice theory (Hardiker and Barker 1981) and beyond the straight jacket of positivist evaluation (Smith 1987; Shaw 1996; Everitt and Hardiker 1996) which is the driving force behind much of the evidence-based social work movement at present. Care Managers may be accused of being 'functionaries' (Hugman 1991) of the community care system, but there is a concept of professionalism which requires the use of a body of knowledge through which care managers, and particularly social workers can evaluate their effectiveness. Such evaluation needs to be critical, reflective and available to practitioners, not mystified and separated in the way that more traditional positivist research does (Smith 1987; Shaw 1996). Research-mindedness in evaluation also needs to avoid some of the simplistic solutions favoured by positivism (Smith 1987; Everitt, Hardiker, Littlewood and Mullender 1992). Service users are unlikely to have the social worker's detailed knowledge of services. Empowerment is the process of matching the user's ability to make sense of their needs and how to meet them, with the worker's knowledge of the effectiveness of potential resources. This is a professional task involving critical and reflective evaluation, part of which would include a request for feedback from users of services or even their participation in the evaluation process.

Like a good general practitioner, the assessor must know what is likely to meet the needs of the assessed person, and set up the contact between service user and service. The effectiveness of the service depends on the sophistication of the worker's knowledge and skills. Referring on to inappropriate services, perhaps by someone following a standard assessment and care packaging formulation is a waste of money (uneconomic), and a misuse of resources (inefficient). It could also seriously affect the interests of the service user (ineffective), although it is the economic and efficiency arguments which are more likely to hold sway within the managerial camp than the effectiveness standard.

The nature of the practice which is informed by this ideology and which is, at the same time, both empowering and protective of vulnerable members of society, is a very sophisticated one indeed. In order to explain it, practice it consistently and evaluate it, such a practice needs an equally sophisticated theoretical framework. Such a framework needs to incorporate the values of social work, which means a practice which reflects the diversity of needs, wishes and experience of those vulnerable and disadvantaged members of society it is intended to serve. The framework, in addition, needs to accept the finite nature of resources and to build the practice of resource prioritisation on such values. There is not one model of assessment mentioned above that balances these criteria. In particular, social work theory is very poor at acknowledging resource scarcity. It may not be surprising, therefore, that social workers feel so deeply the rationing imperative of the managerial approach.

There is a problem of epistemology here too. Assessment takes us into the field of human need, a notoriously difficult area to define in rationalist terms. Doyal and Gough (Doyal and Gough 1991) have provided us with a persuasive theory of human need that claims to establish the universality of human needs, but it remains an area plagued by the doubts of relativism and subjectivism. If social workers are going to steer their way through these swampy lowlands (Schon 1987) then they need to draw upon forms of knowledge that are not straitjacketed by scientific rationalism. Apart from the humanist dimension and empowerment approaches, social work theory provides an epistemology that is built upon a rationalist certainty that is unhelpful to social workers operating in the field of human need. So needs assessment requires not just a practice that draws upon the expressed needs of potential service users, balanced by understanding of the effectiveness of different types of resource, most of which are finite in nature, it also requires an epistemology that accepts the way in which useable knowledge is socially constructed through relationship, by actors using agency. What, in order to enhance the effectiveness of practice is to be the nature of that relationship? Is it to be a traditional professionalism that imposes superior knowledge upon less powerful service users, or will it be one that is participative and actively acknowledges that social relationships are constructed in a context of power?

The Exchange Model of assessment advocated by Smale and his colleagues (Smale et al 1993) is an example of a balanced approach to practice. It starts from the premise that '...all have equally valid perceptions of the problems' (Smale et al 1993; p.7). This gets us away from the professional ownership of assessment advocated in some of the more diagnostic formulations, and task centred case work. The model recognises that practice must seek to establish need whilst at the same time holding 'a view of the resources available to meet them' (Smale et al 1993; p.9). It is important to move beyond narrow service driven practice whilst adopting a framework that recognises there is a link between need and the resources required for their resolution. Concerns that a user focus in needs assessment will open the floodgates of demand on social services department has effectively been disproved by developmental research indicating that service users are only too aware of the finite nature of resources (Beresford and Croft 1993).

The Exchange model is fundamentally humanist in that it recognises that communications involve '...dialogues with people who interpret messages in accordance with their own assumptions and beliefs' (Smale et al 1993; p.11). The dangers of an oppressive practice based on assumption and powerful interest is noted, although the issue of protection of the vulnerable is not ducked. These are not easy areas, they require well trained and sophisticated practitioners reflecting on their actions within a clear system of practice that is congruent with a set of values (Stevenson and Parsloe 1993).

The way the Exchange model advocates 'a move away from focusing on the individual towards the social network...' should avoid the tendency to 'regress to the individualisation of social problems' (Smale et al 1993) which we have noted is so problematic within the medical models above. The importance of community work skills is indicated here. Networking (Trevillion 1992; Beresford and Trevillion 1995; Payne 1993) and community profiling (Hawtin 1992) are, therefore, core skills for exchange practice. The move away from the reification of 'packages of care', and their recognition as being primarily a 'fluid set of human relationships and arrangements' (Smale et al 1993), will prevent the worst excesses of a market oriented practice that turns people into commodities to be brokered, packaged, bought and sold.

The Exchange model could have been supported more fully from some of the theoretical perspectives outlined above. The obvious indebtedness to humanistic traditions within social work could have enhanced its credibility, especially given the balancing realism with which the model addresses the finite nature of resources. Whilst empowerment is a central theme, it might be better enhanced as a model if it pursued its definitions of power more actively.

There is also the potential criticism that the model is idealistic. The sense that the model addresses need within resource constraints but urges practitioners to reflect upon the value base to decisions made is a powerful counter argument. Practitioners using the Exchange model will be working with vulnerable and marginalised people seeking services. The history of their voices not being heard in the application of more procedural or questioning approaches to assessment has already been debated. The Doyal and Gough (1991) concept of autonomy as the universal basis for the meeting of human needs reminds us that, if voice is not heard, there are real dangers that need will not be met in any effective way. Unless assessment on both an individual basis and through the accumulation of these into a wider picture of need adopts the participative approach advocated by the Exchange model, it is unlikely to achieve the expectations of community care policy in providing services to meet the needs of the most vulnerable in our society. If their needs are not in the picture when it comes to making decisions between competing demands, as has happened routinely over the years with the needs of black and other minority ethnic communities, as well as with marginalised groups such as those with dementia and learning difficulties, then the policy is undermined not only within the individual practice of care management but also institutionally. Meeting the needs of the most vulnerable people in our communities is, after all, the political, organisational, managerial and practitioner expectation of community care policy.

The Exchange model does provide this more contemporary approach whilst grasping the nettle of scarce resources. There is also evidence (Stevenson and Parsloe 1993; chapter three of this book) that such practice is extant. Exchange is, however, only a model. The means by which such an approach can be developed is important and the next section argues that the concept of reflection provides a powerful method for establishing a link between theory and practice. In addition, the organisational context in which it can flourish needs to be addressed and this is looked at in greater detail at the end of this chapter. It is also addressed in the following chapters when the second period of fieldwork involving two groups of care managers engaging in co-operative inquiry groups which provided the opportunity for systematic reflective practice is analysed. There is also, in the concluding chapter, some consideration of the concept of learning organisations (Argyris and Schon 1996) and the kind of opportunities this might provide for reflective practice.

As a model which crystallises the usefulness of many aspects of social work theory, even implicitly, as analysed above, the Exchange Model is an example of the purposeful application of theory to inform practice within a clear ethical framework. It has, more recently, been supported by other approaches to assessment within the social work literature such as Middleton (Middleton 1997) who argues for assessment to be seen as a flexible and artistic practice rather than one of applying techniques and rules, and Fisher (Fisher 1997) who sees negotiation as a key activity in assessment and care management which he claims should be, as far as possible, 'an exchange of equally competent partners, rather than a professionally dominated procedure' (Fisher 1997: p. 25). Social work does have a rich enough tradition to be able to provide the essence of such a framework which can be used by social workers to resist agendas in community care practice which appear less concerned for people, and more concerned with the development of successful businesses.

Reflection and the Application of Theory

If policy implementation and managerialism, in their positivist guise, require the certainties of scientific rationalism, then, in the field of needs assessment such approaches are going to struggle to be effective. Needs assessment requires an approach which is at odds with rationalist certainties. That puts social work practice at odds with traditional implementation and managerialist practice. Social work theory, however, as we have noted, is also largely derived from positivist philosophy, seeking forms of knowledge and techniques that are built upon certainty and predictability. It is fair to conclude, therefore, that the confusion of role noted in chapter three is compounded by ambiguity in the epistemological roots to social workers' practice. If social workers resist the techniques of rationalist implementation in its Neo-Taylorist managerial guise, then what can they offer in return? Acting as street level bureaucrats in the Lipsky mould, many social workers are drawing upon a rational social work epistemology that compounds rather than undermines the dominant approach. It is this unreflective use of knowledge in practice that has led to notable failures in meeting expressed need demonstrated in the literature (Ellis 1993; Morris 1995; Harding and Beresford 1996), and noted in chapter three.

In order to operate within the field of needs assessment, what is needed is a flexible and reflective approach to practice, built upon a different epistemology, one that recognises that useable knowledge is constructed by actors in social relationships acting with agency. The Exchange model, built upon a theoretical base of humanism and empowerment provides such a model for practice, but we are still left with the problem of implementation. This is where the notion of reflection as espoused by Schon (Schon 1983; Schon 1987) and developed by others (Boud et al 1985; Boud et al 1993; Gould and Taylor 1996) is important.

Schon's approach to professional knowledge is helpful in developing our understanding of how practitioners such as social workers might operate in what he refers to as the 'swampy lowlands' where 'messy, confusing problems defy technical solution' (Schon 1987; p.3). The personal social services arena would be just such a geographical landscape. Schon, as we have noted above, supports the notion that there is a 'prevailing idea of rigorous professional knowledge' based on technical rationality which is 'an epistemology of practice derived from positivist philosophy' (Schon 1987; p.3). Schon cites the concept of 'artistry' (Schon 1987; p. 13) as the key to effective practice in this environment of 'uncertainty, uniqueness and value conflict' (Schon 1987; p. 6) in much the same way that social work is defined as a creative and artistic endeavour elsewhere (England 1986; Brandon and Jordan 1979).

In order to describe not just what is required of reflective practitioners but also an effective process of learning for them, Schon suggests that it is necessary to develop 'reflection-on-action' (Schon 1987; p. 25), which is the process of thinking back on the knowledge used whilst acting. Schon argues that most of the time this process is 'tacit and spontaneous' (Schon 1987;   p.25). The requirement for reflective practitioners who wish to develop their practice is that they would do this knowingly and openly. The additional, and more complex task of 'reflection-in-action' is the process of thinking *whilst* acting in the same knowing fashion. A more traditional professional will adopt 'rule governed inquiry' (Schon 1987; p. 33) which is fixed and inflexible, whereas the reflective practitioner will adopt more of a developmental learning approach. Schon makes a powerful case for reflection as the most effective way of practising in areas such as needs assessment as I have described it. The principle methodology for practitioners to move from practice using technical rationality to one which adopts a more developmental use of knowledge, is reflection. To become a reflective practitioner is not simple linear learning but a constant process of reflection both on and in practice. This model of learning is supported by other models of cyclical learning (Kolb 1984; Kemmis and McTaggart 1982; McGill and Beaty 1995). Schon posits his 'incompleteness theorem' (Schon 1987; p.255) as the guiding principle - encouraging reflective practitioners to voice their confusion and seek helpful useable knowledge rather than the certainties of technical solutions. This approach to learning and practice development provides us with a method of transforming ill-considered discretion into a more constructive activity which will be looked at in later chapters.

Conclusions

As we leave this largely theoretical chapter it is important to bring the discussion back to a practical note. In order for potentially reflective practitioners to be able to learn to practice in the manner described by Schon, they must be provided with opportunities for reflection, both individually and collectively. This means a managerial or supervisory environment in which there is acceptance that such reflection is a necessary activity. Managerialism which believes that effective practice involves the implementation of rationalist techniques will adopt a management practice that involves checks and controls on the behaviour of practitioners. One guided by the concept of reflection will provide practitioners with individual and collective opportunities for reflection through supervision and team collaboration so that a learning environment can be created.

A management theory informed by empowerment discourse is more likely to achieve the required learning organisation rather than one built upon scientific managerialist beliefs. In the same way, the knowledge base for social work needs to be informed more by Schon's artistry than technical rationality as an epistemology. The congruence between a reflective exchange approach to social work practice, and the concept of the learning organisation (Mintzberg 1989; Senge 1990; Argyris and Schon 1996; Pottage and Evans 1994; Tsang 1997) is quite clear. For both social workers and managers operating in the needs assessment field this could well mean as much unlearning as the gathering of new knowledge.

8 Participation and Action Research - a Coherent Framework for Understanding

Introduction

This chapter provides a continuation of the debate in this part of the book around the epistemological questions. It also acts as a lead in to the next chapter, which deals with the second phase of fieldwork, in which a different methodology to that described in chapter two is tested out. I begin by reiterating the predicament created by the care manager interviews from methodological and authenticity perspectives, noting the epistemological and ontological problems of adopting what was essentially a traditional qualitative approach and analysis. The implication for the research journey was that a new paradigm specifying a new research method was required, and that is what this chapter provides, a description of and justification for the use of what has been termed 'new paradigm research' (Reason and Rowan 1981a; Reason 1988; Reason 1994a; Heron 1996), but is more recently referred to as research within an experiential participative paradigm (Heron and Reason 1997). Co-operative inquiry, one of the methods described within the new paradigm, is described and analysed as a research method in conjunction with our other areas of practice - policy implementation, management and social work.

In the first chapter of this book I include a section in which I dwell for a time on the reflexive journey that this book charts. I indicate the extent to which the early stages were a personal response to the climate or environment in which I was engaged as a researcher - my 'socio-historical location' (Hammersley and Atkinson 1995). This explains the use of the research methodology for the care manager interviews described in chapter three, even if it does not justify the use of a methodology that, upon reflection, was less than comprehensive for addressing the research questions. I was interested in adopting an approach that was enabling but detached when engaging with the interviewees. This was in order to ensure that responses were authentic and not determined by interviewees' position as employees (an organisational response) or as interviewees providing the response that they believed I as interviewer required (researcher effect).

I believe that my practice, using the semi-structured interview approach described and supported by some of the qualitative research methods literature (Foddy 1993; Silverman 1993; Lindlof 1995), was adequate and authentic within the limitations of the methodology, and the sense that I made of what I heard of interest in a traditional academic sense. In written form it was accepted, as a monograph, for publication in a well-respected series (Baldwin 1995). As a piece of traditional qualitative research these interviews have helped me to understand that care managers do act with agency in the way that is described by the bottom-up policy implementation theorists such as Lipsky (1980) and Long and Long (1992) from their constructivist and phenomenological perspectives. This knowledge, with hindsight, is not what makes the research interviews problematic.

What is problematic with chapter three opens a window upon ontological and epistemological issues in research methodology, which dwarf the element of my practice competence. It does not matter how authentic and empowering I was as an interviewer if the issues of ownership and meaning of the knowledge acquired through the interviews are not acknowledged and dealt with. Many academics may have chosen to ignore the non-response to the research report that was promised and provided to the two agencies and interviewees. I was shocked that only three of the 30 interviewees replied to my letter requesting feedback which accompanied the report. Whilst I have since been assured that this is by no means unusual for interviewees who are busy practitioners, it is a matter that still provides food for thought. The sense that I make of this 10% response rate is that the meaning that I had gleaned from the interview transcripts, either held little resonance for them, or, on the other hand, so much that it was too painful to own. I have no way of knowing whether either of these is true or not, but I am left with no foundation for claiming that the knowledge I gained through those interviews made any difference to the lives of the people whom it concerned, even if it helped me in my accumulation of knowledge. If the knowledge was not within the realms of their experience, what is termed 'experiential knowledge' (Reason and Rowan 1981b), then it is not grounded in their actions and its validity is dubious. The knowledge expressed by me in the published monograph (Baldwin 1995) holds the same validity as the key texts analysed in chapter four. It constructs a version of the real world which readers, as actors using agency, can choose to live within, or not.

The knowledge created for the monograph was mine. Useful though it was, that usefulness was limited as far as addressing the main research questions was concerned. It provided information that has persuaded me that care managers as street level bureaucrats can and do skew policy intentions by their interpretation of or resistance to policy directives. This information undermines the claims of rationalists that the correct conditions for implementation will lead implementers towards perfect implementation. There is an additional and implicit question that follows from these arguments. If scientific rationalism is a poor epistemological basis for implementation practice, whether it be political behaviour, management or social work practice, then what are the alternatives that take into account these difficulties? The justification for including this analysis of research methodology is the argument that it provides such an alternative. In addition, if it is put together with alternative perspectives on policy implementation, management and social work practice then we can create a new framework for understanding in all these spheres of action. In its guise as co-operative inquiry this new framework is described in this chapter and explored further, in action, in the next part of the book. It will be argued that co-operative inquiry actually creates opportunities for reflective and critically analytical practice.

Critique of the 'Positivist-Empiricist Approach' (Harre 1981) and the New Paradigm

Harre refers to the 'myth of certainty' (Harre 1981; p.8) in traditional positivist approaches, which is how I would describe the qualitative research methodology that I adopted in the original interviews. There was a sense in which I was attempting to construct an environment in which I could, as a detached researcher, using the correct methods, glean the truth from my research subjects. This approach is based not only on the certainty principle but also on the concept of dualism (Reason 1994a) in which the researcher separates himself (in my case) from the researched just as the knower is separated from the known (Reason 1994a; p.11). Reason speaks of 'these separations on which Western epistemology is founded' and in which intellect is believed to be the 'primary means of knowing' (Reason 1994a; p.12). What happens, we might ask, to the other ways of knowing? What happens to the '*imagined* representation of the world' (Harre 1981; p. 9)? Why this obsession with the rationalist way of making sense? Why ignore affective and behavioural knowing (Reason 1994a; Boud and Walker 1993)?

In a research process which separates the knower from the known, both ontological and epistemological doubts are raised about the knowledge created. Claims to truth from a positivist framework have been weakened from a number of different angles, each of which implies favour for a relativist approach to reality. The dialectical process of reality creation (Freire 1972; quoted in Reason 1994b) argues that we should consider not just the concrete, but also the perception of the concrete. 'We choose our reality and our knowing of it' (Reason 1994b) to this degree. Post-structuralist analysis suggests that it is language which constructs reality (Rojek et al 1988; Potter 1996) and that what counts for knowledge is the 'discourse' that is powerful enough to persuade (Soyland 1994) people of its truth. The reality that defines being in this sense then is limited to a historical and political frame of reference. 'What counts as true knowledge is ostensibly defined by the individual, but what is permitted to count is defined by discourse. What is spoken, and who may speak, are issues of power' (Parker 1989). Humanist psychology also poses a relativist ontology (Reason 1994b; England 1984). Persons, within this framework are viewed as self-defining or self-actualising beings, who 'with help choose how they live their lives' (Reason 1994b; p.325).

This relativism posits a new world view, alternatively referred to as post-modernist (Lyotard 1986; Howe 1994; Parton 1994) or post-enlightenment (Reason 1994b). It is not an individualist world view, however, and human beings are seen as 'co-creating their reality through participation' (Reason 1994b; p. 324). If relationship is also fundamental to the creation of reality, then to adopt a methodology in which the researcher separates himself (in my case) from the researched is to deny and discard that relationship. Ontologically speaking, therefore, the process invalidates the knowledge created, because it does not construct a reality that has meaning for the subjects of the research.

Epistemologically, we encounter similar problems of ownership and meaning. The divisive epistemology of the positivist world view separates the knower from the known and objectifies the subjects of research activity in much the same way that we have seen scientific managerialism and traditional social work theory objectify 'customers', 'consumers' and 'clients', and then treats them as if they were the only reality that needs to be dealt with, rather than very particular constructs of persons, created from very particular forms of knowledge. Explanation is not reality itself, as scientific rationality, with its positivist philosophy, would have us believe. Unless persons are present in the construction of knowledge, unless they participate in the process, the knowledge has no meaning for them. This is a question of power and also, therefore, becomes a matter of politics in not just the research context (Reason and Heron 1995), but in our other areas of interest - management, social work practice and policy implementation.

Rather in the same way that Morgan and Murgatroyd (1994) claim TQM as a new paradigm for management theory, so participative and co-operative research methodology make claims to a new paradigm within research methodology (Reason 1981). Participation is the key to authenticity in this new paradigm for research activity. Orthodox inquiry - the scientific rationalist method - is not adequate or appropriate for studying people as self-determining individuals. The new paradigm is concerned with 'the nature of knowledge rather than the purpose of inquiry' (Reason 1996). Epistemology, then, comes prior to method, with the development of knowledge-in-action being of greater importance than the development of formal theory.

Both Reason and Heron (Heron, J 1981; Reason and Heron 1995; Reason 1994a) suggest 4 forms of knowing which construct an extended epistemology for the new paradigm. All knowing is grounded in *experiential knowledge* which is gained through direct encounter with other people, places and objects. *Practical knowledge* is to do with competence or skill - knowing how to act. *Propositional knowledge* is the formal articulation of other forms of knowledge, and comprises statements or theories that indicate knowledge about something. *Presentational knowledge* is the way we order experiential knowledge, and involves the many ways, through speech, writing, art and movement, that we 'symbolize our sense of their meaning' (Reason and Heron 1994a).

It is propositional knowledge, in terms of formal theoretical concepts that has dominated western academic epistemology within positivist inspired scientific rationality. The dualism, the separation discussed above, means that propositional knowledge has tended not to be grounded in the experiential and practical knowledge of fellow researchers in traditional social science, but instead has been gleaned through inductive or deductive techniques from individuals alienated as objects of research. New paradigm approaches, in recognising the dangers of this separation, require a participative model that ensures that propositional knowledge is grounded in the experience of co-researchers. If we reflect on the position of the care managers interviewed in the original fieldwork, it can be seen that my propositional knowledge gleaned from their words was not fully grounded in their experience, because there was no opportunity to check back in a reflective way the validity of that propositional knowledge. The validity of that knowledge, then, is in great doubt, certainly in the sense that it might make a difference to the *actions* of the people involved. It is only if research is developmental in this way that it can prove to be 'more concerned with developing practice methods in day to day practice ... and address the questions of how practitioners learn and adapt models of practice' (Fisher 1997).

It is the case that some forms of research methodology within the participatory paradigm are more concerned with action by and for oppressed people and this brings the methodology close to the values of contemporary social work. In the case of this particular research journey the issue of voice, which is important within some versions of community care discourse (Wiltshire and Swindon Users' Network 1996; Harding and Beresford 1996; Morris 1994), is restricted more to the marginalised care manager struggling within the managerialist organisation rather than the marginalised and oppressed user of their services. That voice is not heard has far greater effect on the latter group, but it is still a useful concept in understanding and trying to address the feelings of powerlessness that care managers experience in their attempts to develop their practice in what they perceive to be a hostile environment.

Because of the dubious degree of validity in the research interviews described in chapter three, I came to believe that it was essential to use a participative approach for the next research phase. Several approaches have been described within new paradigm research, notably Participative Action Research, Action Inquiry and Co-operative Inquiry (Reason 1994a). It is the latter, co-operative inquiry, that was chosen as the most congruent with the research requirements. The actual process this took is described in chapter nine.   What follows now is a formal description of co-operative inquiry as defined in the work that most completely encapsulates it as a research activity built upon the extended epistemology and ontology described above (Heron 1996).

Co-operative Inquiry as Research Methodology

Co-operative Inquiry treats all those involved in the research process as co-researchers. There is no separation of researcher from researched, even if, as we shall see, individuals within the group adopt different roles at appropriate moments within the research process. Group members act as co-researchers and co-subjects in mutually aiding, reciprocal and authentic relationships. We shall look at how the validity of these relationships and the method is achieved after the process is described. This process follows cycles or phases of reflection and action (Heron 1996) which will be familiar to people who have knowledge of other approaches to adult learning, including individual and organisational learning, that are dynamic in form (Kolb 1984; Boud, Cohen and Walker 1993; Argyris and Schon 1996; McGill and Beaty 1995). There is also congruence with many of the more contemporary approaches to social work methodology, for example self directed groupwork.

In Phase One, co-researchers agree to explore an area of human activity. They agree the questions or propositions that they wish to explore and agree action that would test out this propositional knowledge as well as the systems they will employ for recording. It is principally a phase for propositional knowledge to be used, although some discussion about presentation is clearly important too, so presentational knowledge is also utilised in this phase. Phase Two takes the group members, as co-subjects, into an action stage, in which they test out this propositional knowledge through agreed actions. These actions may be individual or collective, but they should be reflective.   Participants need to adopt an approach, described below as critical subjectivity, that begins to develop some congruence between their action and the propositional knowledge that informs it.   As Reason and Heron put it they should be noticing the 'subtleties of experience' (Reason and Heron 1994a p. 127). At this stage action should not be dominated by prior propositional knowledge in the way perhaps that traditional deductive techniques of hypothesis testing might.

Phase Three is described as 'full immersion' (Reason and Heron 1994a; p.127) in experience. Openness becomes an important concept. Preconceptions or assumptions would be a substantial threat to the authenticity of the learning process at this point. Similarly openness should allow superficial understanding to deepen and be elaborated. The possibility then, of moving away from original preconceptions into unpredicted areas and more creative insights is always present and to be greatly encouraged. Such insights should never be discarded because they do not fit with current propositional knowledge and need, in the next phase to be reflected upon in the co-operative inquiry group and tested out in a process of collaborative learning. The appropriate epistemological concept here is experiential knowing - knowing-in-action. The process of understanding equates closely to Schon's concept of 'reflection-in-action' (Schon 1983).

Phase Four, then, brings the co-researchers back together again for a process of critical reflection, similar, again to one of Schon's concepts - 'reflection-on-action' (Schon 1983). It involves co-researchers sharing what they did in the action and immersion phases and what sense that they made of these stages. This is a point at which new learning is checked against original propositional knowledge and the usefulness of that form of knowing verified against experiential knowledge employed in the action and immersion phases. Prior knowledge may be altered or discarded completely, or there may be a feeling that it needs to be further tested, perhaps in a slightly different way in the next cycle of action and reflection. Effectively Phase Four feeds into a repeat of Phase One in which propositions are restated and further action for testing propositions is decided upon. These phases are then repeated in a number of iterative cycles until either a predetermined point of review is reached, or, through mutual agreement, it is decided that original propositions are adapted to a point where possibilities for further testing are exhausted.

Validity in Co-operative Inquiry

It is an important part of participative action research, of which co-operative inquiry is a part, to separate it from reflection and action within an action research model (Kemmis and McTaggart 1982; Carr and Kemmis 1983; McNiff 1992; McGill and Beaty 1995). Action research as a model is very closely associated with co-operative inquiry methodologically, but it is usually associated with research carried out by practitioners, sometimes in collaboration with one another, but into their own practice. Whilst this is close to the model that was tested out and is written up in the next chapter, the difference is that action research is still often carried out by a group of professionals (teachers, in much of the literature) upon others. So although there is the conceptualisation of constructing meaning in collaboration within action research, there is still the tendency to adopt a model of separation of the researcher from others who are being researched. This was an eventuality which I was keen to avoid for the second phase of my fieldwork, given my experiences following the interviews. In addition action research misses the concept of 'critical subjectivity' (Reason and Heron 1995; Heron 1996). This form of thinking is the method by which co-researchers 'develop their critical awareness of the theories and ideas they bring to their action in the world' (Reason and Heron 1995; p.124). We have already noted that research within an experiential participative paradigm is not one built upon the one reality of scientific rationality, even if it may involve a process of exploring truth. There is an acceptance of the different ways in which sense can be made of experience, but it also the case that co-operative inquiry accepts that researchers may have good reasons for being 'resistant to noticing inadequacies in the idea that the experiential grounding reveals' (Heron 1996 p.146). Critical subjectivity is a form of reflexiveness that creates in co-researchers an awareness of biased thinking such as unaware projections (Reason and Heron 1995; p. 149) or collusion. Reality is not an absolute but a process. 'As we choose and co-create our world, our knowledge can develop this quality' (Reason and Heron 1995; p.124). It is this quality and practice of critical subjectivity that is the cornerstone to validity in the research methodology.

There is a similarity between co-operative inquiry and the less well defined approach to organisational learning that Argyris and Schon (1996) refer to as the 'theory-of-action approach'. They define organisational learning as occurring when individuals within an organisation experience a problem and then enquire into it on the organisation's behalf. Action and reflection which then shifts their understanding of organisational phenomena and results in them 'restructuring their activities' (Argyris and Schon 1996: p. 16), or changing their behaviour, so as to bring outcomes and expectations into greater congruence, is a process which will change an organisations 'theory-in-use' (Argyris and Schon 1996: p. 16). This explicit shift in theory-in-use, rather than the tacit changes that happen in less reflective fashion in organisations is what constructs it as a learning organisation. Argyris and Schon do not duck the issue of values and learning. It is not a case of any learning being a 'good thing'. Critical judgement is certainly implied within the concept of reflection on the importance of value in learning, although there is not the same adherence to critical subjectivity as there is with co-operative inquiry. The focus on learning as cyclical and affecting behavioural outcomes is an important part of both approaches. As Argyris and Schon argue, the process of enquiry affects outcome because it can affect the individual's construction of meaning within the organisation if they wish it so to do. Whilst the 'theory-of-action approach' may be less well formulated than co-operative inquiry, it is a methodology that is tied in with organisational learning, which brings it closer to my intentions, rather than co-operative inquiry which could involve a group of co-researchers inquiring into similar issues but from very different backgrounds. The learning in co-operative inquiry is mutual, but, in the Argyris and Schon approach it is organisational too. For the care managers I was intending to work with, their role and position within their organisation was a crucial issue, as will become apparent.

The appropriately structured and rigorous approach to validity in co-operative inquiry is one of the factors which made it a useful model for me to follow. Co-operative Inquiry moves beyond the use and abuse of the term validity in the epistemology and politics of positivist research (Heron 1996). Heron believes that outcomes of co-operative inquiry are valid 'if they are well-grounded in the forms of knowing which support them' (Heron 1996; p.57). The validity of forms of knowing depends on the degree to which they are 'well-grounded in the procedures adopted to free them from distortion' (Heron 1996; p.57) Heron claims that there are special inquiry skills and procedures involved in this process of ensuring validity (Reason and Rowan 1981b; Heron 1996). The skills involved are built upon concepts within humanistic psychology, and would be instantly recognisable, for instance, to anyone knowledgeable in Rogerian techniques of counselling and psychotherapy (Rogers 1951). One of these skills is authentic presence which is based upon the concept of empathy - a process of understanding the other's experience. This was an approach that I tried hard to achieve in the first set of interviews through my interpersonal skills, although I can accept now that the concept of shared meaning was missing, which made it less likely that the relationship and what flowed from them were 'authentic' in the way Heron describes. 'Imaginal openness' (Heron 1996; p. 58) is the skill of being receptive to meaning from an intuitive perspective. In the process of mutual learning it is important to be able to imagine what different meaning to our own a particular experience might have for a colleague in the group setting. If one were to start from a view that there is only one reality and a different one is a mistaken one, then clearly it is going to be difficult to construct a participative form of learning. To understand colleague's perception through their perspective requires this concept of imaginal openness, so that mutual learning can take place. The congruence with good, anti-oppressive practice in social work will not go amiss for those conversant with practice debates in this area. It is a very similar process to that defined in good practice in the art of assessment in, for instance, care management (Smale et al 1993; Middleton 1997). To imagine achieving an approach such as this in the space of a one hour interview is impossible. Such validity could really only be achieved through relationship in a trusting environment over time. Such luxuries are not available in traditional interviews such as those described in chapter three. 'Bracketing' (Heron 1996: p.58) is the skill of managing the concepts - the propositional forms of knowledge - that we use to make sense of experience. Managing in this sense means recognising that we are using them, and critically evaluating their usefulness in the process of making sense. Bracketing is, therefore, a key part of critical subjectivity. 'Reframing' (Heron 1996: p.59) is another skill in this process of managing concepts. Defining an idea in a different way is a skill that tests out assumptions and allows a degree of mutual analysis in any given circumstance. Whilst I was able to reflect on the use of concepts whilst making sense of research interviews in the earlier fieldwork, there is little doubt that such an approach is far easier to construct over a period of time in collaboration with others in a co-operative inquiry group. Again, reframing, is a practice familiar to social work practitioners making sense of the lives of service users in the assessment process. 'Dynamic congruence' (Heron 1996: p.59) is a form of practical knowing, in which the purpose of behaviour, its value and motives can be judged and revealed. It is referred to as dynamic because such congruence is not likely to exist at a fixed point in time but will develop as the process of learning progresses through its iterative process. Judgements about the validity of knowledge needs to progress at the same rate at which the learning process advances and develops. Again a process of research that passes through cycles of reflection and action is more likely to be valid in this sense than one based on a snapshot of 'how it is' at a given moment. 'Emotional competence' (Heron 1996; p.59) acknowledges the affective element in learning and knowledge accumulation within new paradigm research. This is very close to Boud's concept of 'attending to feelings' (Boud and Walker 1993). Early experience and social conditioning are two ways in which knowledge can become distorted and inauthentic. Being able to recognise when this process of distortion is happening within a co-operative inquiry group is an essential skill for at least some of the participants to possess. As well as being able to note this emotional content in others' actions, it is important also to develop a degree of 'non-attachment' (Heron 1996: p.59) so as not to invest personal identity and emotional security in the action phase of research cycling. It will be seen, in the next chapter, that this practice that is crucial to ensuring validity was hard enough to maintain within the comparative safety of a co-operative inquiry group. It is even harder for me to know what kind of affective responses that I created through the interviews in the first piece of fieldwork. It is very possible that concerns and anxieties were raised that led to a less than candid response to the questions I was asking. How would I know? Last of the skills Heron lists is 'self-transcending intentionality' (Heron 1996; p.59) which involves being able to reflect upon different forms of understanding which may help offer explanation even whilst in the process of action. We have already noted the similarity with Schon's 'reflection-in-action' (Schon 1983).

The validity procedures which have been developed for Co-operative Inquiry are designed to try and free the process of inquiry and learning from the 'distortion of uncritical subjectivity' (Heron 1996: p. 59). In planning the phases of research in a co-operative inquiry, these validity procedures need to be actively programmed in. Research cycling, which effectively describes the methodological process is a form of validity procedure itself. Cycling through reflection and action takes the co-operative group through experiential and reflective forms of knowing in a process of knowledge refinement leading to increasingly authentic and shared forms of knowledge. Again this notion of cycling is congruent with other approaches to adult (Kolb 1984) and organisational (Tsang 1997) learning. Divergence and convergence is the process by which a group would explore the issue at hand both from a specific and then a general perspective. This could happen within one cycle or could be divergent in one cycle and convergent in the next. This process increases the opportunities for the issues in question to be explored in the different ways of knowing. There is a process here of dialectic - alternating between the particular and the more general in pursuit of congruence and agreement. Reflection and action is also one of the actions which defines the methodological process and is central to the validity claims. Heron's claim is that 'reflective and experiential forms of knowing refine each other through cycling to and fro' (Heron 1996: p.60). There is, in this practice, an important issue of balance between reflection and action. Too much of the one would potentially favour one form of knowing above another, which would undermine the validity of the outcome. The central technique for assuring validity is a simple devil's advocate role which is ascribed, at different times in the whole process, to all members of the group or perhaps to a particular individual in a discussion. This devil's advocacy is required to test out whether there is any uncritical subjectivity distorting the creation of knowledge in the co-operative inquiry group. The devil's advocate (in the nicest possible way) is there to expose such behaviour as avoidance, collusion, fixation, false assumption and lack of rigour in applying other validity procedures.

Chaos and order is a more recent addition to co-operative inquiry validity procedures and acknowledges the usefulness of a dialectical process of alternating between chaos and order that occurs when members of an inquiry group are being truly open in their thinking. Sinking into chaotic thinking can, for people raised within Western modes of learning be a worrying process. For co-operative inquiry, chaos holds the opportunities for creativity not present in the more ordered processes of scientific rationalist inquiry. This process of descent into chaos can, however be an anxiety provoking process and may conjure reactions from participants such as 'unaware projection' and 'inauthentic collaboration' (Heron 1996: p. 60/61), so techniques for dealing with anxiety and stress within the co-operative mode of operating is an essential part of maintaining validity at a high level.

These techniques, of research cycling and validity, are descriptive of the research methodology but should not, in any sense, be seen as constricting what should be a flexible and exploratory approach within a co-operative framework. The openness required to ensure that learning happens in the cycles of action and reflection would be completely destroyed by any absolute and rigid application of the techniques. Heron admits considerable concerns that co-operative inquiry within what he terms the 'Apollonian' distinction - a 'more rational, linear, systematic, controlling and explicit approach' (Heron 1996; p. 45) - could be just as dangerous as a completely 'imaginal, expressive, spiralling, diffuse, impromptu, and tacit approach' (Heron 1996; p.46) which he defines as 'Dionysian', using Neitzsche's distinction. At either extreme - rather like the chaos and order dialectic - co-operative inquiry could either solidify into objectified knowledge or scatter into incoherence. The importance of role within the group is then of great importance and is something that needs to be planned for in the initial phase of a co-operative inquiry group's lifetime.

Roles and Relationships

If co-operative inquiry concerns the creation of useable knowledge through the process of relationship, then it is important to address role within inquiry groups. We have already looked at some of these issues in relation to validity procedures. The devil's advocate is an important role to fulfil but there are others. In order to maximise the opportunities for collaborative inquiry, it is essential that all members of the group are able to participate to their full potential. Inclusion and influence for all is the key as 'each person's agency is fundamentally honoured' (Reason and Heron 1995; p.135). Group facilitation, then, is an important role to be cultivated by one or all group members. Knowledge and skill in group processes (Brown 1992; Preston-Shoot 1987) is a key to this, although it is not claimed as a professional task, but one that 'ordinary people' can develop (Heron 1996: p.134). A co-operative inquiry group could have a specific person as facilitator, or it could be a task that is shared within the group. It is, however, important to establish the ground-rules at an early stage in the group's life, and monitor and review progress at intervals.

Group development theory informs us of the normative stages of group development. The initial stage, after forming, is one of anxiety and sometimes conflict. Whilst the devil's advocate role is important to ensure that problems are not avoided, but dealt with honestly and head on, it is also important that there is some form of leadership in order that the group can be guided through these difficult times. Leadership is not necessarily perceived of in the traditional sense of one person taking a dominant role. It can be an alternating system shared intuitively within the group, or a mutual shared role. The role for leadership is to maintain group cohesiveness through difficult periods, and ensure that direction is maintained. Direction, again, is not the absolute that more traditional approaches might advocate. We have already looked at the importance of chaos as a creative force. Direction could, at some stages be very haphazard. It may take collective leadership to create enough mutual courage to travel down an unknown and potentially dangerous path.

Support and nurturing are other roles that needs to be fulfilled in co-operative inquiry groups. The reason for this is that they are learning groups and learning, when it is successful, is very often stressful and painful (Baldwin 1996c). Learning is a process of creating new knowledge and new understanding, but it never occurs within a vacuum, but always within a relationship to prior knowledge. Very often, then, learning means the negation of previously held understanding. If the area of inquiry is one that group members feel close to and have invested much emotional and intellectual energy in, then to have to unlearn keenly held knowledge, beliefs or values can be painful, at the least. At its most acute, such learning can undermine individual or group beliefs about themselves, knowledge that they may well feel is self-defining. Under these circumstances, paying attention to individual and group health, in its broadest sense is a central role for group maintenance. This role is often performed by one or two members who recognise and expose such difficulties. It is possible to build such a role into the group processes by taking time out for evaluation, and then making use of other forms of support, perhaps completely separate activities that encourage cohesion without the pressure of addressing the issues at hand (diversionary approach) or by holding specific group sessions to look at process, perhaps asking an outside facilitator to enable this process should it have become stuck (therapeutic approach).

Linkages - A New Framework for Understanding the Research Questions

Co-operative Inquiry was the methodology chosen to follow up investigations into the research questions. These questions were *What are the limitations   to successful policy implementation?* and, more specifically, *Are policy intentions undermined by frontline or 'street level' implementers?* The developmental question is *Are there different forms of implementation that take into account and include the influence of other participants?*. The first stage of fieldwork, for all the shortcomings of the methodology, established for me that the limitations are, to a substantial degree, the result of the activities of frontline practitioners acting with agency as Street Level Bureaucrats, largely in defiance of rationalist attempts to impose forms of knowledge and ways of acting upon their practice. If street level implementers' actions are important in defining policy outcomes then the knowledge that informs their actions needs to be congruent with the knowledge that informs the policy intentions. Knowledge possession, however, as we have seen, is not an absolute, but a creative process. At its most effective, it needs to be creative within participatory and reflective relationships. It requires ownership of meaning before knowledge is accepted and makes a difference to the actions of individuals or collective groups. This is the case when we are referring to the collection and dissemination of data for research purposes, and that is why a new research paradigm has been argued for. If a participative research methodology is not employed, then the danger is that research replicates the problems that we have already noted in relation to policy implementation and managerial practice when they attempt the imposition of policy through technocratic means, and then wonder why social workers resist. Interestingly, exactly the same process is noted in the practice of social workers when they employ scientific rationalist practices with service users (Stenson 1993). Resistance and a reduction in effectiveness and positive outcome is the result.

In order for authentic participation to occur, self-defining people need to be present in the processes by which useable and powerful knowledge is created. Managerialism, through the processes of eligibility and prioritisation, define consumers of welfare services. Policy directives (Social Services Inspectorate 1991a and 1991b) use similarly objectifying language such as packages of care to define interpersonal relationships. Social work too, in traditional theoretical concepts objectifies and depersonalise clients within a medical discourse. Lastly we have traditional positivist research which separates and classifies objects of research. We are looking here to move beyond this traditional, scientific rationalist conceptualisation of individual people which objectifies, and, within new right ideology, commodifies individuals as workers (units of production) and consumers (units of consumption).

What this book argues is a unified and integrated model for practice within research, policy implementation, management and social work practice, that is built upon a participative world view (Reason 1995;

Heron 1996). Such a world view needs to adopt a critical approach to the construction of knowledge within its participative framework, recognising the need for self-defining individuals to be present in the process of knowledge creation if such useable knowledge is to have meaning for them. Co-operative inquiry may require, or result in, taking sides against more powerful creators of knowledge (Reason 1996). We have already seen, in chapter four, that Community Care is a reality that has been created by persuasive discourse, but that there is scope for the deconstruction of such powerful forms of knowledge and the substitution of others. Community Care holds within itself the seeds of its own transformation, particularly because the political discourse has been constructed to try and speak to different constituents, including those less powerful in the whole - that is firstly frontline practitioners - the professionals - and secondly service users, who are clearly bottom of the pile when it comes to the power to change the dominant ethos of resource control. There is much evidence within the service user literature (Beresford and Croft 1993, Evans 1997; Harding and Beresford 1996) that collaborative effort can produce knowledge that is a powerful opposition to dominant thinking. Service users cannot produce more resources, apart from that which exists within their own individual and collective strengths, but they can change the way in which thinking about formal resource distribution is conducted. The fear often expressed that service users would ask for the earth has generally proved incorrect (Beresford and Croft 1993). What service users want is the opportunity to participate in the process of decision-making about resources that can fundamentally affect their quality of life. Where they are allowed to do this, the evidence is that they are happier with the quality of service received (Beresford and Croft 1993; Harding and Beresford 1996). Practitioners too are often marginalised by organisations that place decision-making in the hands of senior managers and/or elected representatives. Even within TQM the empowerment only follows from the creation of the mission statement which is constructed by senior managers (Morgan and Murgatroyd 1994). A more participative approach between politicians, managers, social workers and service users, it is argued, would be more likely to produce outcomes, in terms of knowledge for action, that would hold greater meaning for all, and would, therefore more likely be owned by them and make a difference *in practice.*

In policy implementation terms this means adopting an approach that is less concerned with techniques for approaching 'perfect' implementation, and more with participative and democratic forms of organisational structure. Policy implementation is affected by the activities of street level implementers, so if they are not a part of the process formally, they are likely to skew it informally through the more or less unreflective use of their discretion. Management, in the 1990s, is the principal tool, within the organisation of social welfare services, for implementing policy directives. Management that is informed by scientific techniques is likely to be resisted far more by street level implementers who have had no part in the construction of the relevant knowledge that informs implementation practice, than a more democratic and inclusive approach. TQM and Mintzberg-type learning organisations are the nearest we have to a form of knowledge that approaches management practice in this way. There is a hangover from the New Right obsession with management in the 1980s that still projects management as the key task, rather than one which requires managers to collaborate with others in a process of knowledge creation and practice development. When this essentialism begins to fade, as it is within much of the more contemporary literature on learning organisations (Argyris and Schon 1996; Pottage and Evans 1994) there will be an opportunity to match management theory and policy implementation theory with (in our illustrative example of care management) social work theory, to construct a unified conceptual framework that is inclusive and participative. As far as research is concerned with the creation of useable knowledge, it is very close to these other areas of practice. In order to test out this integrated conceptual framework, we can investigate the success of an experiment in two co-operative inquiry groups run by the author, with groups of social workers who have a care management role in a local authority Social Services Department. Whilst this is limited as an all-embracing experiment, it is in the nature of such innovative work that it is small scale. The lessons need to be learnt, and the methods re-tried and tested.

9 Care Managers Investigate their own Practice

Introduction

In engaging with care managers in co-operative inquiry I was attempting to do a number of things. The first was to construct a situation in which I could glean from care managers the current state of practice as far as their role in the continuing implementation of community care policy was concerned. This would provide evidence to compare with that from the first set of interviews, and address the research questions about limitations to policy implementation and the role of street level implementers. In addition, I was interested in exploring the possibilities for utilising co-operative inquiry to develop practice that might, in a small way address some of the problems of more traditional forms of implementation. This meant, effectively, the testing out of co-operative inquiry as a research methodology which involves learning and practice development. Recognising that social worlds are constructed by actors in relationship with one another, this approach seemed an appropriate way to investigate with street level bureaucrats as they played their part in constructing community care policy. Finally, in the spirit of co-operative inquiry as a participative venture, I was keen to respond to the interests of the group members with whom I was to engage. This, I believed, held the promise of revealing other issues that had not been apparent prior to this.

The process started by an offer being made to the training manager of a Social Services Department to feed back the findings from the original interviews, and asking participants, in a workshop situation, to address themselves to the question of how far these findings were 'true for us?'. This was a form of inquiry, in itself, that had been tried and tested as a form of research dissemination in the past (DHSS 1985). At this stage it had also been negotiated that an offer would be made to practitioners who were involved in the workshop, that they could engage with me as facilitator in one or more co-operative inquiry groups for the purposes outlined above. There were two workshops, attended by a total of twenty social workers and one first line manager. The social workers were all involved in a role similar to that carried out by care managers described in the first set of interviews. They were, effectively, care managers, carrying out an assessment, care planning, monitoring and review role for adult care services provision. The manager was responsible for a team of social workers fulfilling this role in a hospital setting.

There was agreement that the findings from the interviews were still a matter of concern to care managers. In particular, resource constraint still has too great an influence on assessment practice, with service users getting little in the way of comprehensive assessments of their needs that was not distorted by resource availability. Social workers still resist the creation of unreal expectations in vulnerable service users by adopting a purely needs-led approach. There was some feeling that the bureaucracy of care management - the 'instruments of assessment' - were now more familiar to social workers and less intrusive into practice. However, there were still some areas where there was concern that the bureaucratic process, along with resource constraint, was stifling the use of professional discretion, effectively managing out social work as a service available to users. This was apparently the issue of greatest concern to practitioners, partly because it undermines their role, by marginalising the knowledge, skills and values that underpin their practice. In addition, this process of marginalising social work as a service was, in participants' view, denying users access to a service that could prevent the eventual imposition of more restrictive resources such as residential care. It was, participants felt, an inefficient and ineffective process that ought to be reversed. Social work was seen as a preventive service that was being marginalised by an obsession with more formalised types of service, and most notably, very expensive residential care. There was complete agreement with the original finding that targeting those in greatest need was an ineffective way of providing service as it frequently means waiting until informal support networks fail and then providing formal services either in crisis, or a position of unacceptable risk, as judged against rigid eligibility criteria. This was another example of ways in which organisational processes undermine professional social work practice.

The two workshops ended with a description of co-operative inquiry as a way of investigating and working upon the problems that had been identified and I offered to convene one or more groups to engage in a co-operative inquiry process. The result of this offer was that two groups were formed.   One was a team of five hospital based social workers (Hospital Group) who had been a team for some time and were keen to engage as a group to investigate their very particular circumstances, as well as more general issues.   The other group (Community Group) was formed from a more disparate collection of social workers, some of whom worked together in already established teams and some who were in different and separate teams. This group numbered eight in total.   The two groups met separately, and there was early agreement that it would be helpful if I was to take a role as convenor. Both groups met a total of eight times over a six month period, and the group sessions were concluded a few months later with a workshop in which both groups met together and with managers from the local authority to review the learning that had been done across both groups.

The question needs to be asked to what extent these two groups were co-operative inquiry groups in the way described in the previous chapter. At the point of evaluation, at the last of the meetings, it was agreed in both groups that the process had involved a participative and co-operative approach. Members of both groups were involved in decisions about what would be the areas for investigation and of the methods that would be used to explore, in both action and reflection stages. Both groups progressed through cycles of action and reflection - eight in all - using a variety of methods for investigating the action being taken, and forms of recording to be used in the action phase. As far as recording the reflective meetings was concerned, I was taken up on my offer to record meetings, on the understanding that the notes were always a draft and needed to be read and approved by all group members before being agreed as an appropriate record. There were occasions when this principle was put into action and notes were changed as a result of discussions, so it was not just a vacuous exercise. In hindsight, however, it is clear that an audio-recording of the group discussions would have yielded more of the detail, individuality and intimacy of the mutual discussions than written recordings based on contemporaneous notes. I am not able, as I was with the first set of interviews to offer actual quotations in this chapter. I feel this is regrettable, but it was not felt to be an appropriate or necessary form of recording at the time of group formation. There was a great deal of general anxiety and suspicion in both groups about the nature of what they were being *allowed* to do in engaging in these co-operative inquiry groups. Meeting together outside of team boundaries to discuss work is not permitted in this local authority Social Services Department, as in many others, so an exception was being made in this instance. An audio recording of their discussions was perhaps viewed as a more permanent record of their discussions which might have placed them in jeopardy. I was sensitive to their request for using written recording - ostensibly in my words - as it distanced them slightly from the recording.

The role of facilitation was offered to me by both groups. This was appropriate as I was the outsider in a sense, the only group member who was not directly involved in the role that they were investigating. This meant that I could be convenor of the group, facilitate group discussion and play a valuable role as 'devil's advocate'. I was not the only person to do this in either group nor did my role as facilitator mean that I was in an exclusive leadership role. These roles were, at different times, also adopted by others in both groups. The groups were, then, participative and democratic. With the particular exception of the recording issue, my view is that they were co-operative inquiry groups in the sense defined by Heron (Heron 1996).

Both groups completed eight cycles of action and reflection, as indicated above. Attendance at group meetings was very high. We agreed in both groups that they should be closed, in terms of future involvement by others, but inclusive in terms of always ensuring that all members were present before proceeding. There was one occasion on which one member was absent, because he was unwell at the last minute. Apart from that every session was fully attended and we did not have to cancel any sessions. The level of commitment and involvement was thus very high. At the first meeting there was an 'idea-storming' session, in which possible areas for exploration were recorded, discussed and then selected for investigation. Both groups soon realised that there was enormous room for manoeuvre, holding a potential for co-operative inquiry to be fed with potent areas of investigation for far into the future. Decisions were made about what action could be taken in the interim period and how it could be recorded prior to reconvening for the first reflective meeting.

We had reached a point at which the co-operative inquiry groups had been formed within the broad framework that I had set out at the time of the initial workshops. The specific areas for exploration were chosen by the groups, and it was at this stage that the democratic process of group decision-making was in evidence. It is very interesting that the two groups came up with broadly similar areas for investigation, and that they were both largely driven by anxiety about their performance as social workers within the authority. In hindsight it is easy and perhaps pertinent to make the connection between the anxieties that fuelled their desire to explore consistency of practice and their concerns about audio recording. When the issue of stability of employment in this authority which is discussed later in this chapter is added, then a web of issues around anxiety and security begins to emerge. There is an element of post hoc rationalisation in this analysis, but, as will be seen below, we did make some of the connections at the time, especially recognising the need to acknowledge and address anxieties as potentially powerful blocks to learning and practice development (Boud and Walker 1993). If sensitivity to this affective climate resulted in the loss of opportunity to record the richness of the voice of participants then that is unfortunate. I do not believe that it conflicts with my analysis that these were co-operative inquiry groups, nor do I think that it undermines, in any great sense, the validity of the inquiries.

The question of why the groups chose this particular area to focus on rather than some of the others that they listed in the idea-storming process is an interesting one. Looking at the notes from the original discussions two things are revealed. Firstly the anxiety that motivated the choice was argued as important to deal with and not ignore. If it was not tackled at this stage we believed that it could sit silently in the room providing an environment that would undermine commitment to mutual learning. Secondly it was felt that the focus on practice issues that they had some day-to-day control over was a more practical proposal than looking at more intangible areas such as resource deficits, which was another of the areas discussed as holding a potential for exploration. Not only would the chosen area of investigation be more possible, they also held out, in our mood of early day optimism, the chance of achieving successful outcome. We did not want to travel down any gloomy dead-ends.

The aims of these cycles of action and reflection were much the same for both myself and other participants. They were interested in seeing what the possibilities were for developing their practice over a period of time, in what they understood to be the policy context for their role as care managers, but also utilising their social work practice in the process. There was, particularly in the Community Group, some scepticism that there would be many opportunities for using their professionals skills in this way. Professional discretion was believed to be in serious decline if not already killed off by the new role of care management which had been imposed by a management agenda which was ruled by resource constraint rather than service provision. I was interested in seeing to what extent the process of inquiry could investigate areas such as the use of professional knowledge in a discretionary way, and, I was keen to see how the conjunction of their social work skills with the new role of care management might be the catalyst for the creation of new knowledge informing a new practice. From chapters four and seven it can be noted that the Exchange model (Smale et al 1993) of practice in assessment and care management was drawing on the best of social work knowledge, skills and values and a new empowering model of resource allocation to present a new paradigm for adult care practice. How achievable was this practice, using co-operative inquiry as the motivating force?

The Process of Co-operative Inquiry

The groups met separately, usually for an hour and a half at a time. We ensured that the time was uninterrupted, and all members were present, something achieved on every occasion except once. The first meetings for both groups established ground-rules around group processes, roles, confidentiality and whether the group was to be open or closed. We also discussed the manner in which we were to relate to one another, for example avoiding personal comments, but forming a mutual agreement that problematic issues would always be raised and addressed in the group, rather than discussed outside. These discussions, which are very similar to those suggested in the group-work literature (e.g. Brown 1994) as good practice when establishing cohesive groups that are intended to perform effectively over time, were agreed as of crucial importance. Establishing such ground-rules at the earliest opportunity makes it more likely that future unforeseen eventualities that might block group processes and group learning will be dealt with effectively.

As indicated above, anxiety was recognised as a prime area for investigation in the 'idea-storming' session in the initial meetings of both groups. The principal anxiety for both groups was identified as lack of consistency between individual team members and between differing teams. How, inquirers wondered, would they know, as agency employees, what the practice requirements were? This question was a surprise, given the existence of what might be considered fairly comprehensive guidance documents. What was apparent to both groups, quite independently, was that interpretation of guidance was different between individual workers and across teams. It was this differentiation that created the anxiety.

Hospital Group Discussions

The Hospital Group decided to tackle this issue by focusing on a very specific piece of bureaucratic procedure to see what the differences and similarities of practice were. The form chosen was the one that had to be signed by a potential service user, with the purpose of gaining consent for the department, in the person of the social worker, to contact third parties to assist the process of assessment. This consent was seen by the agency as good practice in that it reflected a process of partnership. Social workers in the Hospital Group were concerned that, for some people they interviewed, requesting a signature on this document was a threatening, disorientating or even oppressive practice. When they felt this to be the case, they did not ask for a signature, even though they knew they were *supposed* to. It was an example of the ethos of community care policy in a practical exercise but also the use of discretion and was thus a worthy focus of investigation from both angles. It would allow the group to investigate the extent to which policy was being undermined by the use of their discretionary practice. In addition it would provide an opportunity for both convergent inquiry (the very specific case of this form's completion) and divergent thinking (transferring this learning from the specific to the more general issue of the use of discretion).

The process that was followed from this initial identification was to devise a technique of investigation and recording. Every time that one of the forms *should* have been completed in the period intervening reflective group meetings, participants were to record the circumstances and the reason why they did or did not ask service users to sign the form. In effect they were required to justify their actions, both to themselves and to their peers in the co-operative inquiry group. This provided an opportunity to both reflect-in-action ('why am I practising like this now?') and, at a later time to reflect-on-action ('why did I ask *that* person to sign the form but not *this* one?'). This was an interesting example of Schon's reflective process of learning and developing practice, in action (Schon 1987). This process was followed for three consecutive cycles of action and reflection. At the third meeting one member of the group, acting as a 'devil's advocate' quite rightly questioned what the purpose was of continuing this exercise. This allowed the group to diverge from the immediate task and look at the wider implications.

The main result of this challenge was that we entered into a fascinating inquiry into the nature of intuition. As facilitator I asked group members how they knew when it was the *right* moment to ask someone to sign the form and when not. The first response was "I know intuitively when it is right" - "I get a gut feeling that it is not right with this patient". We then proceeded to deconstruct the concept of intuition, by continually asking *how* the individual knows, and *where* that knowledge comes from. We identified the sources of knowledge, the theoretical perspectives, the social work values, and the skills, as well as the assumptions and prejudices that often combine to make us act in one way rather than another. All this jumble of knowledge - experiential, propositional, practical and presentational - had been combining together to inform practice in a generally unreflective way prior to the group's engagement in the co-operative inquiry process. Every time we got to the bottom of intuition, defining it and describing it, we were still left with something indefinable, which was labelled intuition again! "I just knew that I shouldn't push her on signing the form." I described what I saw as a 'threshold technique' intuitively (at best) or unreflectively (at worst) being employed by group members. At some point they were able to recognise that a particular individual met some undefined criteria that meant they could cope with being asked to complete the required paperwork. The service user was then asked to sign the form. How did they know that they had crossed that threshold? What knowledge, what skills, were being employed to assist that decision? An exercise was developed, with a system of recording attached, to enable group members to go into the next action phase and engage in utilising the threshold technique. This technique, plus the recording process used in the inquiry cycles, encouraged the social workers to maximise opportunities for participative practice. As a result, there was an increase in the numbers of forms signed without a consequent increase in service user or worker anxiety.

On meeting again we found we had even more material to help in the definition of intuitive knowledge, sifting out the propositions from the practical and experiential ways of knowing. Intuitive knowing was seen as an important aspect of creative understanding, although we were agreed that it needed to be recognised and reflected upon, because there were substantial dangers involved in not reflecting on use of knowledge in the way that we had started to do overtly. This process of reflection in and upon action was enabling group members to differentiate the use of knowledge that was informed by the sorts of participatory and empowering values that they espoused in theory, from the more assumptive or stereotypical practice that they recognised occurred sometimes if they were *not* engaged in such a reflective process. Recognition of this potential for basing practice on assumption created considerable anxiety which needed to be dealt with through group processes, particularly for some of the newer members of the team who had not been qualified for so long. It seemed, in this small group, that experience was a factor that increased confidence to at least some degree. 'Return to experience' (Boud and Walker 1993) was a key to this process of developing reflection-in-action. Whenever new ways of understanding were created in the group they were tested out and incorporated into behaviour that was subsequently confirmed as appropriate or adapted accordingly.   For all of them, however, it was anxiety provoking to recognise the potential for acting in potentially discriminatory ways. Discrimination is such a negative factor in contemporary social work ethos that identification of such a tendency in one's own practice can create considerable anxiety. Some of this anxiety was recorded in the first set of interviews.

The importance of reflection in and upon action had thus been established as a key to the maintenance of, and the continuing development of good practice in the light of new circumstances - such as the introduction of new policy or procedure.   When, the group asked themselves, did they have such opportunities to reflect upon their actions? How, they continued, could they instil the discipline within their actions to ensure that they practised reflection whilst actually engaged in relationship with service users? The co-operative inquiry group was providing such an opportunity, but what would happen when it finished?

The answer to this question was raised in conjunction with another line of thought in the Hospital Group. This involved the group's concerns (shared with the Community Group) that social work as a form of knowledge and values was being marginalised by the introduction of care management into their department. As with the care managers in the previous fieldwork interviews, they recognised that social work was often the only service that could be provided to prevent informal supports from breaking down and more restrictive services such as residential care becoming inevitable. How was it possible then, to protect the room that they might have for providing good quality assessments, develop a preventative service, and ensure that they had opportunities for reflection and practice development? This led us into exploration of the usefulness of different forms of workload relief, but also into the realms of management and supervision. Group members recognised that supervision was an important arena for both reflection and decision-making around workload relief. They also recognised that they relied upon their manager to give them the time and space for good quality supervision which included feedback on their practice. This was one way, outside of the co-operative inquiry that they might establish some overview of their practice to ensure consistency. How to encourage their manager to provide this service to them as a team became a focus for one cycle of action and reflection. They also explored the possibilities for mutual aid in providing support when they felt stressed, and space for mutual reflection upon work they were engaged in. Through these processes the team gradually developed their own individual and collective techniques for replicating the most useful aspects of the co-operative inquiry in anticipation of its closure after the agreed six month period.

Community Group Discussions

So how did the Community Group fare? Their focus for investigation was not dissimilar to the Hospital Group, a piece of procedure which they believed they were engaging with inconsistently. The inconsistency was creating anxiety and they wanted to look at their practice in order to try and develop the *right* way of doing it. By the right way, they meant a combination of agency procedural consistency along with a consistency in practice as informed by what they agreed were good values in social work. On investigating the minutiae of their own practice and then sharing on reflection, this group were most surprised to discover the degree of discretion that was available to them. Most group members were convinced that the introduction of care management had effectively managed out opportunities for using professional discretion in social work. They were somewhat anxious to find that they were engaged in discretionary practice in an unreflective way. It was far less easy, therefore, to blame inconsistencies on organisational processes, or lack of resources from area to area. Much of it came down to their own actions. The group owned this learning and then engaged with it over a period of time, exploring the ways in which they could develop their practice, bringing agency policy and professional practice into closer proximity.

The way the Community Group proceeded was mainly through sharing of individual practice in a supportive environment. Everyone was given the time to talk about a recent piece of work, and questioned supportively but in a challenging way so as to deconstruct, to the greatest degree possible, the sources of knowledge that were informing their practice. This was a different process but led to a similar outcome as the Hospital Group. We had similar discussions around the use of intuition and what this was, although it proved far harder for this group to avoid the debate around the influence of organisational constraints and resource shortfall. Opportunities for emotional off-loading and support tended to be more necessary in this group, probably because it was a less cohesive group than the Hospital Group who were already a team in their own right prior to their formation as a co-operative inquiry group. Having said this, the nature of organisational influence resulted in both groups, at different times, having to use up one whole session reflecting on the way re-organisation was affecting them personally and collectively. There was talk of redundancies and re-application for their jobs as well as the dispersal of their immediate team managers during the lifetime of the groups, which brought understandably high levels of anxiety into group processes. It is an indication of the two groups' commitment to their own practice development that this context of change and uncertainty did not deflect them more often from their investigative project.

In a sense the Community Group was more vulnerable. It was harder for them to engage to the same degree as the Hospital Group, although the level and sophistication of discussion around practice development was still generally impressive. The co-operative inquiry approach provided them with an opportunity for actively learning, mutually creating knowledge and understanding that could be tested out and incorporated into their practice. One member remarked on how he used the group, in the action phases of the cycles, to enable him to 'reflect-in-action'. He did this by asking himself "what would the group think of me doing this, saying that?" when he was actually engaged in relationship with service users.

One of the main areas for exploration in the Community Group, with their greater degree of interest in organisational processes, was the way that they experienced what they termed 'buffeting' and how they might resist it. Buffeting was what happened to their practice as a result of organisational changes and resource management processes. Buffeting reduced their scope for professional discretion and determined the course of action in assessment and care planning with individual service users to a substantial degree. This involved similar discussions to the Hospital Group about methods for recognising and enhancing discretion and pushing back the more negative aspects of managerial and organisational control. Both groups recognised that there were opportunities, as I had learnt from the original interviews, for developing methods of using bureaucratic procedures to achieve practice development, and equality of access to services for users. On occasions this meant the use of discretion to redefine such procedures, and plan how they would defend this in the face of managerial hostility. One of the areas of learning, as shall be seen below, was a recognition of the importance and usefulness of the organisation's mission statement, drawn up, in good TQM fashion, by senior management and approved by elected representatives. What group members realised was that procedural requirements were very often apparently at odds with this mission statement, and this gave them the opportunity to resist the managerial definition of practice in favour of one which was actually more in tune with not only the mission statement, but also social work values. The most notable example of this was the separation of the ethos of quality public services, in the mission statement, from that of resource management, which seemed to be the principal thrust of managerial activity during the lifetime of the co-operative inquiry group. As indicated above, this was the main source of the 'buffeting' which group members believed prevented them from engaging in positive social work practice.

The Validity of the Process

What can be added to this about the use of validity skills and procedures? The concept of 'critical subjectivity' (Heron 1996) has been argued as the key to validity in co-operative inquiry. We have already listed the skills for ensuring validity in the previous chapter. There was, I believe, a high degree of authentic presence in both groups, based upon the sort of empathy that develops from a mutual understanding about the pressures involved in a task such as social work. Members of both groups already had a primary level of understanding of the other's experience. 'Imaginal openness' (Heron 1996; p. 58), it will be remembered is the skill of being receptive to meaning from an intuitive perspective. We have seen how this concept of intuition was explored in detail. Neither of the two groups rejected the importance of intuitive thinking, indeed, the process of deconstructing the knowledge base to practice validated a range of different ways of making sense of practice, including intuition which was accepted as an important force for creativity. 'Bracketing' (Heron 1996; p.58) and 're-framing' (Heron 1996; p.59) are the skills of managing the propositional forms of knowledge used to make sense of experience in the action phase of the research cycling. Managing in this sense meant recognising the forms of knowledge that were being used as people are using them, and critically evaluating their usefulness in the process of making sense. These are key aspects of critical subjectivity and, I believe, were actively engaged in during both group's lifetime, even if reflection involved a struggle on occasions. 'Self-transcending intentionality' (Heron 1996; p.59) which requires being able to reflect upon different forms of understanding which may help offer explanation even whilst in the process of action was noted above as similar to Schon's 'reflection-in-action' (Schon 1987). This was another skill of validity development that was engaged in during the groups' cycles of action and reflection. We discussed ground-rules at length in the first session of each group and made it quite clear that respect for different perspectives should be fundamental part of the values of these co-operative inquiry groups. That there was little evidence of different perspectives on issues displayed may say much for the congruence in social workers' ways of making sense of their circumstances. It may also say something about the safety in which we conducted our business. As the person who had perhaps the least to lose by exploring different angles on issues, I am not persuaded that there was too much convergence into comfort zones. Whilst validity as the reliability of our findings over time may have been less rigorous than more traditional approaches, the level of authenticity in our discussions was generally at a high level. It will be remembered that it has been argued that authenticity is more important than reliability (Silverman 1993) in research within this paradigm.

Research cycling is argued as the key technique for ensuring validity in that cycles of reflection and action take the co-operative group through experiential and reflective forms of knowing in a process of knowledge refinement leading to increasingly authentic and shared forms of knowledge (Heron 1996). This process and that of divergence and convergence facilitated the groups' exploration of the issues at hand both from a specific and then a general perspective. It is important to remember the issue of balance between reflection and action, and convergence and divergence to ensure that there is a corresponding balance in the development of forms of knowing. This balance was lost in the Hospital Group at one point in favour of a more action orientated process. Luckily there was a brave enough devil's advocate on hand to ensure that this imbalance did not persist!

I am not sure to what degree the groups allowed any process of dialectic between chaos and order in group processes. I suspect that we kept much of the discussions at a fairly safe level. I do not believe that this resulted in the inquiry being inauthentic. If there had been more of a collective mind to explore chaotic ideas then we may have learnt more. The sensitivity of the area of practice being investigated, and the degree of anxiety around job security for most participants probably excluded this possibility.

Learning from these Co-operative Inquiry Groups

There now follows the curious process in which all the good intentions described above are undermined as the author articulates his own version of the outcome of the learning in the two groups! At some point we all have to own our learning, and what follows is my version. As we have seen there is much in the literature (Heron 1996) about validity, and the safeguards that have been developed and were described in the previous section ensured a high degree of congruence between what is now said and what was agreed collectively in the groups. The next section of this chapter is based closely and carefully upon a paper that I wrote for the two groups and senior managers within the Social Services Department to summarise the outcomes of the two groups. This was shared with group members who required some changes to the paper, but were in broad agreement. This section remains, however, my version, which others may or may not fully agree with.

The two major themes that have evolved from these inquiries take us back to the heart of Lipsky's (1980) arguments. Discretion and accountability are the two headings under which most of the discussion and learning can be filed. The two groups found themselves addressing the question of what accountability means if it is to enhance positive use of discretion rather than the more negative and tacit use of discretion which was creating anxiety for practitioners. The anxiety was particularly acute as participants feared that their practice was inconsistent both with agency policy and with colleagues. They were also concerned that inconsistency could result in an inequitable or even discriminatory service being provided. This would undermine their commitment to social work values which urge a practice that avoids the replication of organisational and societal disadvantage for many service users. It will be noted that the problem of ambiguity in Community Care policy exposed in chapter four remains a potent issue for care managers. Whilst policy from central Government, often supported by Social Services Department guidance, continues to speak the language of managerialism, then social workers feel they have something that they need to resist. This managerialism is revealed in two ways. Firstly by an emphasis on resource management as the prime purpose of organisational practice and secondly through the application of techniques of neo-Taylorist scientific management such as eligibility criteria and priority matrices. The chapter ends, however, on a note of nascent optimism, following the final joint workshop held between the two Inquiry Groups, at which the managers present spoke with some passion about the importance of the managerial role in enabling the use of professional discretion and empowering staff. They even apologised for the lack of success in achieving this aim during a period of general Local Government re-organisation, followed by internal changes designed to meet major resource shortfalls.

1. The Search for Consistency in Bureaucratic Procedures and the use of Social Work Knowledge, Values and Skills

There were a minority of interviewees in the first fieldwork event who were able to describe bureaucratic procedures as a way of providing equality of opportunity for potential service users. This was a major area of learning for the two groups, particularly if these procedures (notably the forms) were used through the medium of a participatory relationship and were not an administrative application. In order to ensure that this difference was consistently acknowledged and maintained, the co-operative inquiry groups recognised that opportunities for reflection (Schon 1987; Gould and Taylor 1996) on the use of knowledge skills and values was essential. The normative places for such reflection are in supervision and team discussion. Because of pressures of work and management style, these opportunities are not always available to practitioners. The co-operative inquiry created such an opportunity, thus exposing what participants had been missing hitherto.

The inquiry groups gave participants the opportunity to reflect on their use of discretion in relationship with service users in a positive and developmental way. There was an ownership of poor practice as participants reflected on their prior use of discretion and then devised methods for testing out more positive approaches, returning after periods of time to reflect within the group on their success. As this process of action, reflection and learning proceeded, so we learnt that prior belief in the death of discretion in the face of coercive bureaucracy was (to paraphrase Mark Twain!) premature.

Intuition was seen as an important concept in analysing the use of discretion. The groups attempted to deconstruct intuition, reflecting on the way in which it can reveal assumptions, based on prior knowledge and experience. It became apparent that such intuition could dictate practice and result in inconsistency and discrimination. The importance of reflection to evaluate sources of knowledge, skills and values that inform practice was revealed only too clearly. The groups were left, however, with a deep commitment to the importance of intuition as one of the major sources of creativity in practice. This is a view supported heavily by the work of writers such as England and Jordan (England 1986; Jordan 1984; Jordan 1979; Brandon and Jordan 1979) who also equate intuition with creativity within a humanistic paradigm.

Bureaucratic procedures, during these inquiries, shifted from being symbols of managerial excess to opportunities for resistance to that alien culture. They were seen as models of good practice which provide practitioners with the justification for a needs-led, user-focused and participative practice which was in opposition to the resource management position that was felt to be the driving force behind managerial practice. The groups started to think about developments beyond the good practice defined by the forms, looking, for instance, at more sophisticated ways of seeking service user feedback, and considering ways in which services might become more relevant to people from minority ethnic communities who are often denied access to such services as a result of racism (CCETSW 1991b).

This approach allowed participants to get beyond the anxiety created by resource shortfall, and to develop practice that reflected their set of values rather than managerialist concerns. There was also a strenuous argument that these social work values are more congruent with the Authority's mission statement of service than the managerialism they were resisting. One example of this is the social model of disability (Oliver 1996; Morris 1991), which they felt was a key value that informed their practice. The resource management angle which employed techniques of targeting and prioritisation are, for these groups, forms of labelling that are completely at odds with the social model. Most participants had been on much heralded training courses provided by the Authority which emphasised the social model of disability. To expose this organisational dichotomy - the values the organisation espouse at one point placed in opposition to what they propose at another - is a powerful form of deconstruction, which effectively destabilises organisational practices when they are so clearly anomalous.

Practice, it was learnt, has two extremes, both of which have the potential to create very negative outcomes. At one end it can be ruled by unreflective discretion which leads to inconsistent or discriminatory practice. At the other end it can become unthinkingly routine, leading to unimaginative or stereotypical responses to individual need.   The recognition of a need for balance between these two poles gave participants the analytical tool for their reflective practice that was so helpful and developmental within these groups. As long as it is operated within a reflective environment, discretion is a powerful force for developmental practice. Future opportunities for reflection are still required. It is a perpetual project. The worth of reflection and the tools required have been established for these individuals within the co-operative inquiry groups.

2. Accountability through Enhancing Collaboration and Partnership

There were three ways in which partnership could be seen to operate and enhance the positive development of practice.
*   creating forms of good practice in collaboration with colleagues in multi-disciplinary networks within and outside the Department. This is a long term process which requires opportunities for individual and collective reflection to avoid collusion and negativity (e.g. stereotyping of service users). There was concern expressed that organisational changes, which were fragmenting teams and separating colleagues from different disciplines, was resulting in a management-driven threat to Government policy on multi-disciplinary assessment.
*   with service users, in order to manage the tension between being a professional and an agency worker. There was much reflection in these groups about the way that partnership reveals power relationships which then marginalise some service users through, for instance, the processes of disability or colour-blindness. Partnership,

and the use of advocacy, were seen as opportunities for resistance to resource management as the dominant discourse and the substitution of a concept of service as the motivation for practice.

• with managers in the department. There was a feeling of marginalisation within the department, and a desire to be involved in organisational processes. Personal responsibility in this was acknowledged and, for instance, some work was done to enhance the degree to which service deficit was recorded. Since the completion of the group sessions, it has been accepted by management that greater participation by staff with considerable knowledge and experience could be an effective way of maintaining a process of service development. This is particularly important in the light of increasing organisational fragmentation, internal competition and marginalisation of professional concerns. This is not a new battle, but is now understood by participants in a more sophisticated way which moves beyond 'they-ought-to-do-something-about-it' syndrome.

3. Accountability, Management and Control

Lipsky's concerns about coercive forms of control and the resulting development of unreflective forms of discretion was important in learning that opportunities for reflection, evaluation and feedback through developmental and inclusive forms of management were essential. The groups' understanding developed over the period of the inquiry, and a number of practice responses to this issue of management were attempted. The lack of opportunities for reflection was a key problem area. Workload management to create more opportunities for this activity have been actually implemented in one of the teams concerned. The other result in this more empowering form of management was to free up time, within workloads, for the provision of social work *as a service* to users. This is particularly important in a climate of acute resource shortfall when practitioners recognise that they are often all that is available to vulnerable and needy service users. They need to create time outside of processing assessments if some vulnerable people are going to receive any service at all.

Despite the concerns about resource management and control, there remained anxiety about the degree of consistency of practice across the Authority. How, the groups asked themselves, do we know what the Department expects of us? Are we doing it *right*? The groups noted the potential gap between normative definition of a good assessment, and what was actually happening at the practice level. The gap, it was believed, is filled by resource constraints, which pressurised workers into practice which they knew was not prescribed either by policy intentions or social work values. The most obvious example was the pressure to assess according to resource availability, not needs, to avoid creating unreal expectations in service users. This, it will be remembered, was a routine practice by many of the care managers interviewed in the first set of interviews. There remains considerable pressure, some of it self-imposed, upon social workers to adopt this approach, rather than enter into the challenge of developing the highly sophisticated practice of collaborative needs-based assessments with service users.

Group members tried hard to commit themselves to greater use of service deficit recording as their responsibility in the process of developing responsive services. This is extremely hard to do in the face of organisational blocks to creative packages of care such as the linking of budgets to current service provision. The 'net cost policy' which should allow workers to gain access to the money that they *would* have spent on residential care, to put together community alternatives, is almost completely overwhelmed by these blocks, leaving no room for creative use of resources to meet individual need. There are dual responsibilities here, and group members, as a result of these deliberations, understand the separation of their role from that of the Authority much better.

4. Care Management - a Professional or Administrative Role?

This is a subject that reflects an area of great interest in the literature (Payne 1995; Shepperd 1995). Wondering whether it was a professional or administrative task did not detain either of the two inquiry groups for long. Their day-to-day immersion in the complexities of other people's lives left them in no doubt that assessment and care management are sophisticated tasks requiring a degree of knowledge and skill beyond administrative technique. This approach is supported by Fisher who demonstrates 'how difficult and demanding is good social work practice in community care' (Fisher 1997; p.26). The complexity of the concept of need, which is almost brushed aside in the Social Services Inspectorate guidance (SSI 1991a; SSI 1991b), the problems of remaining needs-led, mentioned above, and the exhortation to multi-disciplinarity and the development of a user-led practice are some examples of the arguments that care management is a professional rather than an administrative practice, although this is not the place to go into the complicated arguments around the conceptual differences noted elsewhere. In the face of this complexity, discretion is not a block to policy implementation but a necessary tool for practice. What makes it different in practice, however, was believed to be the emphasis in professional social work on reflection during and after practice (Schon 1984 and 1987). The use of reflection as a form of evaluation within contemporary professional practice can be seen as quite different to outcome evaluation in resource management terms.

Reflections and Conclusions

The purpose of co-operative inquiry is the mutual creation of owned and useable knowledge. In reflecting on the co-operative inquiries above, it has been seen that this purpose can be fulfilled by social workers investigating their practice in a participative framework. Both co-operative inquiry groups established new areas of understanding, some of them previously unrealised insights and others resulting from revisiting and adapting formerly held knowledge. Unlike the knowledge created from the interviews at the first stage, this knowledge held meaning for the co-researchers which they were able to own and adopt in their practice. The creation of knowledge in these groups thus had an effect on behaviour in the way that might be expected from an approach that is congruent with models of cyclical learning (Kolb 1984) and reflective practice (Schon 1984; Boud and Walker 1993; Gould and Taylor 1996). As a system of investigation co-operative inquiry has proved more effective than traditional qualitative approaches in facilitating the production of owned and useable knowledge. As street level implementers, the individuals in both groups recognised that they are able to use their discretion to influence the introduction of policy in certain ways. This influence can be either positive or negative, but they will be unable to differentiate the nature of the influence unless they adopt a critical reflective approach to their use of discretion in practice. Co-operative inquiry, as a research methodology, and as a form of active learning can be successful in facilitating a process of learning in which participants can incorporate different forms of knowledge into their practice.

It is important to question whether these conclusions are over-idealistic. It could be argued that the co-operative inquiries were a one-off which will not, in the long term, change anything in social services organisations which are still wedded to the kind of managerialist techniques discussed elsewhere in this book. The counter arguments are, firstly, that the co-operative inquiry was presented as an experiment in the possibilities for engaging in reflection and learning for developmental practice. No more was claimed for the groups than that. As an experiment, however, I conclude that it has proved highly successful in revealing the possibilities for a dynamic and developmental use of discretion within social work practice where practitioners are given the opportunity to reflect upon their practice, especially in a collaborative fashion as they have been in this case. Such opportunities do not only provide positive benefits. They also set up an environment of dynamic and reflective use of discretion which is likely to force out the negative results of ill-considered or unreflective discretion which is revealed elsewhere in this book from empirical evidence as well as being argued conceptually as normative within the street level bureaucrats' modus operandi. Such experiments do require further investigation through replication in different settings to test out their effectiveness in reducing policy implementation deficit, as argued in this book.

The second point concerns the practical nature of the developments that have come from the groups' reflections. Workload management systems were explored as a method of freeing up social workers' time to engage in more preventative work. Such space would also create the potential for more opportunities for reflective evaluation such as that provided in the co-operative inquiries. This was one practical outcome of the inquiries that required no additional resources and could be achieved despite organisational constraints.

In addition, work was done on exploring effective ways of persuading first line managers to offer dynamic and developmental supervision which would also replicate, on an individual basis, opportunities for reflection established collectively through the co-operative inquiry groups. The third practical development resulted in participants becoming more actively engaged in seeking opportunities already available for participative reflection and developmental thinking, for example within training provided by the authority. Again, these developments required no additional resources as they were already provided.

Lastly, in this list of practical developments that could be accommodated within prevailing organisational parameters, and which were not resource dependent, participants agreed to make better use of the participatory opportunities already available within the organisation. These included the recording of unmet need which was, indeed, an agency requirement. Participants realised the potential for adding the data collected through the accumulation of their day-to-day assessments into the process of service development and strategic decision-making by engaging in this practice that they had previously felt to be a waste of their time. To do so was not only potentially effective, it also employed them in action that hitherto they had not been able to see the purpose of, and which, through their non-engagement, had added to their anxieties. There were also other opportunities for participation offered by management in the organisation. Following debate within the co-operative inquiry groups and with the senior managers after their completion, prior scepticism about these opportunities gave way to a new feeling that it was important to take such opportunities as they were presented. It was too easy to dismiss such opportunities as tokenistic. To brand them as such and then ignore them was to turn such appraisal into a self-fulfilling prophecy.

It is not too difficult to note the congruence between the outcome from these co-operative inquiry groups, with the other strands - policy implementation, management technique and social work practice - which have been addressed in this book. The co-operative inquiry approach revealed the degree to which participative investigation and learning can produce positive outcomes that are more consistent with policy intentions than coercive approaches to policy implementation and practice development based on the certainty principle of scientific rationality. The final chapter takes up these issues in a much broader analysis of co-operative inquiry and the participative action orientation to learning and development, reflecting upon the micro-arena of these two groups and imagining what might be learnt in the broader areas of organisational process and policy implementation.

10 Policy, Discretion and Learning in Organisations

Understanding Policy Implementation - Rationalism or Social Construction?

So what are the implications for future practice in policy implementation, management, social work practice, and prospective research? We need to acknowledge the limitations of the co-operative inquiry groups as an experiment in the construction of useable knowledge, but I do make a claim that there is evidence from this research that scientific rationalism as a form of knowledge to direct policy implementation, managerial and social work practice is far less helpful than more participative forms of development, based on a social constructivist epistemology for both understanding the complexities of implementing social welfare policy and in the action of implementation. This addresses our primary questions posed at the outset of this book. Practitioners, as street level bureaucrats, can and do use their discretion or agency as actors within the community care arena to practice in ways which has the effect of constructing policy which is not congruent with original policy intentions. That policy is socially constructed in this way requires the policy analyst to adopt an evaluative approach to policy implementation that assumes the importance of all actors in constructing policy. Whilst accepting that the responsibility for policy initiation lies at the top of organisations, an authoritarian imposition of policy is unlikely to be successful. This undermines the scientific rationalist approach to policy analysis and policy implementation that was looked at in chapter two.

The reason for this is that a social welfare policy such as Community Care is about the nature of human relationships. Human beings construct their day-to-day reality through such relationships. Ontologically, human existence is a process of constructing a continually unfolding reality. Such an ontological position requires an epistemology that addresses the creation of knowledge, and does not engage in a search for reality. Both positions construct reality, rather than respond to a reality believed to pre-exist and about which continuing inquiry will make us more and more certain. Human beings have the capacity to create and recreate their being from moment to moment, so any form of human activity that is predicated on the certainty of outcome in any situation involving human relationships is going to be uncertain in its validity. 'Authenticity', it will be remembered, 'is more important than reliability' (Silverman 1993). My concern about the methodology for the interviews in the first piece of fieldwork is far less to do with its accuracy in relation to a reality external to the participants than its meaning within the every day lives of those participants. Scientific rationality that assumes the facts and seeks to establish what they are in order to establish rules for action whose outcomes can be measured, is not an appropriate philosophical basis for inquiry into human action. Research which is collaborative, involves an honest sharing of interests and active participation is more likely to lead to acceptance by those it concerns and changes in their behaviour (Smith 1987).

Policy Implementation and Human Agency - the Power of Discretion

In policy implementation terms, scientific rationality assumes that correct procedures will determine outcomes which can be predicted and then measured. Human agency would be one of those variables which is open to manipulation and prediction. What the research discussed in this book has demonstrated is considerable support for a theoretical position within policy implementation that asserts the importance of human agency in constructing policy despite the intentions of top level implementers. Evidence of this human agency is revealed in the discretionary practice demonstrated in both stages of fieldwork described in this book. It is backed up from other sources of empirical and theoretical work (Lipsky 1980; Stewart and Ransom 1988; Ellis 1993). Discretion by street level implementers such as care managers, whether it be of the unbridled form, or reflected upon in the way that was described in the previous chapter, is itself evidence of the potential for human agency even in highly technocratic managerial organisations. The possibilities for such agency were the same in all three organisations in which empirical work was carried out. It made little difference whether there was a well-organised rationalist managerial technology in place or not. Discretion will happen because human beings will create their own reality through relationship.

The other issue for human agency in the form of discretion and in the context of policy implementation is about effectiveness. Here too we can argue that discretion is essential as well as inevitable. If community care is about the political process of organising services to meet the needs of vulnerable human beings (Malin 1994; Means and Smith 1994) , then it is also about the management of human relationships (Smale et al 1993; Middleton 1997). Because human behaviour is complex and unpredictable, and involves communication to make sense of other people's lives, very often across cultural divides, then a flexible and reflective approach is essential to ensure effectiveness. There are no certainties to discover through the use of rationalist techniques. Each truth needs to be created, through the medium of relationship and skills in communication through a 'constant set of approximations' (England 1985), each one checked out along the way to ensure that understanding assumed, and knowledge created, is agreed between those involved. Professional discretion in the process of making sense of other peoples' lives, which is what assessment involves, is thus not just inevitable but essential.

If professional discretion is inevitable and essential for the implementation of a human services policy such as Community Care, then what should be the nature of such discretion and how can it be developed to meet the intentions of policy in terms of outcome and value? Discretion in its unbridled and unreflective formulation, as described by Lipsky (Lipsky 1980) and revealed in chapter three of this book, is not a form of practice that is likely to be in any sense helpful to the construction of knowledge that could help care managers and service users know how to act when involved in assessing needs and implementing care plans. We have seen how such use of discretion has the potential to predicate a traditional professionalism that assumes and imposes suitable knowledge on a given situation, rather than engaging in a process of mutual learning and understanding. Positive and developmental use of discretion will have other qualities. The first of these is that it should be *reflective.* Reflection is the process, it will be remembered from chapter one, by which we return to experience (Boud and Walker 1993). We build our understanding and knowledge upon that experience in the way described by Heron (Heron 1996). The authenticity of propositional knowledge - the formal theory which we act upon - is judged by the extent to which it is built upon experiential knowledge. Reflection also encourages us to attend to our feelings (Boud and Walker 1993) so should include affective learning too. Reflection in the co-operative inquiry groups meant learning from the anxiety created through practice as much as anything else. To have sought certainty to eradicate that anxiety would have meant ignoring the confusion of the world of community care and trying to side-step feelings rather than deal with them. Discretionary behaviour based on unacknowledged feelings can be very dangerous. Reflection is also the process through which critical subjectivity can be ensured. We are not talking here of uncritical learning, and values within what is learnt and the forms of knowledge that inform practice need to be made clear (Argyris and Schon 1996). Reflection is, finally, about re-evaluating experience (Boud and Walker 1993) so is as much about a process as an outcome. Reflection is a fundamental part of creative learning (Kolb 1984), in which we move in a cyclical process from the creation of knowledge to understanding. We saw in the last chapter how social workers used reflection to make sense of what they termed intuition. This was a very good example of people working co-operatively to create a more exposed form of knowledge upon which they could act from the murky waters of careless intuition and indiscriminate assumption that existed before and which held such dangers for those vulnerable service users whose construction as 'clients' with 'needs' was at the mercy of unreflective care managers. It is these processes which differentiate the practitioners that were involved in the co-operative inquiry groups from Lipsky's street level bureaucrats. It is in this sense that the participatory forms of knowing and social action espoused in this book take us beyond the Lipsky critique of discretion in practice.

In chapter one, I made a claim to being a reflexive researcher, so being *reflexive* too, is an important part of discretion. Reflexiveness requires a practitioner to be aware of the social and historical location in which their practice exists. We have seen in chapter four how Community Care has been constructed by powerful forms of knowledge in a historical and social framework. Each practitioner's practice is also a combination of such constructs, enacted through human agency. In order to be honest about the social-historical context in which practice takes place, practitioners need to be reflexive, show themselves to themselves. This is a process of authentication, which is essential in cross-cultural communication. To fail, for instance, to recognise the effect of communication between a non-disabled social worker and a disabled service user, or a white male manager with a black woman practitioner, is to disregard the context of power in which relationships are constructed, and the potential for miscommunication that consequently exists.

Discretion is a powerful force in a domain such as social work practice. We have seen the way in which it can determine outcomes that may well not be in the interests of services users within care management, for example with service-led assessments rather than needs-led assessment within a service user focus. If discretion is not used in *participation* with service users, carers, colleagues from within and beyond the practitioner's agency, and with the wider community, then it is unlikely to be developmental and effective. Participation, in this sense, means authentic relationships, constructed for the purpose of mutual understanding as much as to achieve some particular outcome. Participation is a process of coming together which acknowledges differences of perspective but endeavours to reach agreement on how to act by pooling those sources of knowledge and creating an agreed collective strategy for action. That is why it is important to be equally as aware of process as outcome in the evaluation of practice (Smith 1987). It would be a failure of partnership to exclude any individual's perspective in the construction of knowledge for action. Practitioners in community care have the power, through their use of discretion, to determine the degree of authenticity in this concept of partnership. Although such power may be limited in their dealings with other professionals, for instance a service user's General Practitioner, with service users themselves, they can, and do, as we have seen, routinely exclude less powerful individuals from the process of participation in activities like assessment which fundamentally affect their quality of life.

This exclusion is interesting when it is considered that social workers experience the same feelings of exclusion within their own organisations. Within Social Services Departments it is managers who have the power of discretion to influence the degree of participation engaged in by street level implementers. There is a process of mirroring here. If, for instance, an assessment of a service user's needs is to be authentic, that is, if it is to mean something to all the people involved, and be a valid basis upon which to act, then all the parties to the process need to participate in the way described above. If a service user is denied the opportunity to participate in this manner, then they will not be present as subjects in the process by which useable knowledge is created. It will not have meaning for them, and will not be a valid assessment upon which to act. It is more likely to construct a basis upon which to resist, in any of the ways people know how when faced with oppressive behaviour by more powerful actors. It is resistance to a non-participative management that causes social workers as street level bureaucrats to behave in the ways that we have seen described in other sections of this book. Participation, then, is for everyone, and defines a new approach to practice in the different areas of interest that we have covered - policy implementation, management, social work practice and research. Participation is a buzz word within social work and community care, as it is in many other arenas. What I believe has been demonstrated here is a way of getting beyond the emptiness of the buzz. Policy and management too often assumes that saying things often enough, and with increasing sanctions attached will lead to desired outcomes. What is claimed in this book is a method, built upon a well argued and epistemologically sound theory that will enable participation - in policy implementation, in management and in social work practice - to become more of a way of life in organisations that work with some of the most marginalised and vulnerable people within our society. Participation is not an event but a process, a long road down which it will always (to quote the Chinese proverb) be better to travel hopefully than to arrive. Arrival would signify the end of the struggle to balance the competing interests and perspectives of participants with differing sources of power to draw upon as they create and re-create their existence.

Policy Implementation and Discourse

We saw in chapter four how human agency can be understood to occur within the context of more or less powerful forms of knowledge, which can be termed discourses. Within Community Care we have noted a number of competing discourses, the most powerful of which, in terms of influencing the organisational processes of policy implementation, has been managerialism, supported by a new right political agenda. The discourse of social work is less influential in the face of this managerialism, although, as we have also seen, the differentiation of these forms of knowledge is not as simple as might first be assumed. When we look behind the facade of managerialism, for instance, we can see that there are different forms of management knowledge, which, according to some writers (Morgan and Murgatroyd 1994), indicate different paradigms. Social work knowledge too has developed a new paradigm according to Adams (Adams 1996). The differentiation with a more traditional approach is argued as the separation between scientific rationalist and social constructivist epistemologies that inform the separate paradigms. So although social workers have been seen to resist managerialism, by the use of their agency through discretion, they are not averse to employing forms of knowledge from social work theory which are based on a similar view of the potential for the expert pursuit and capture of certainty in human affairs.

To try and comprehend this environment of policy implementation, in which competing discourses provide us with alternative forms of knowledge to construct Community Care, it is essential to adopt a critical approach. Emergent awareness of discourse and the power that it wields in determining our real worlds, is a process of deconstruction. This process both exposes the nature of the discourse and reveals the alternatives that could replace it as powerful and persuasive rhetoric. In Community Care we have noted that new right political rhetoric has constructed a version of community care that is concerned with providing opportunities for consumers to be involved in making choices within a free market for welfare. This rhetoric has been supported by the organisational reconstruction of Social Services Departments into purchasing and providing sections, the managerial practices of targeting, prioritising in order to control scarce welfare resources, and control of key staff through changes to working practices and, to some degree, de-professionalisation. This reconstruction of human services has been largely dishonest in its failure to acknowledge the limitations of resource availability, preferring distribution to become apparent through market processes, rather than by exposing shortfalls. To deconstruct the discourse of 'choice' and expose its limitations - 'choice equals constraint' (chapter four) - is to construct in its place an alternative discourse of service user involvement which is built upon a liberationist view of participation and involvement (Freire 1972). In this case we are not objectifying and labelling service users as potential welfare consumers, but perceiving them as self-determining individuals requiring help and support to ordain their own futures. This discourse celebrates difference, it does not objectify and classify in the way that more traditional approaches to assessment practice do. It enables self-determination by creating space for individual and collective empowerment. It is honest and open about resource constraint, and views distribution as a collective responsibility that can be negotiated rather than determined.

Policy Implementation and Future Participation

We have arrived at a point where policy implementation is being pictured as a battle ground for competing forms of understanding, different ways of making sense of what is, by all accounts, a confusing world. Community Care is a confusing world partly because it is an expensive one and the political processes of resource distribution are therefore acute and contested. It is also a confusing world because the welfare needs of a modern state are a battle ground of value too. There is no longer a consensus (if there ever was), for instance, that society *must* care for older people through state intervention. There is a powerful modern ideology that says people should look after themselves. That there is a vigorous debate going on at present about the degree to which pension providers were wrong to persuade people to move from mutual pension funds to individual and personal pensions, is an indication of a possible shift from the powerful individualism that constructed welfare policy in the 80s and early 90s. Differing beliefs about welfare create a world of confusion. Finally, Community Care is a confusing world because it is made up of people. To objectify Community Care, as rationalist policy theory does, is to construct it outside the experience of many of the stakeholders who are involved. It is these stakeholders who construct Community Care on a day-to-day basis, acting as more or less free agents in relationship with one another. Relationships are messy confusing affairs. Community Care is thus confusing because people's behaviour is unpredictable, and because relationships between people are unpredictable.

People who give a damn about the implementation of Community Care policy are interested in ensuring that it possesses some form of structure so that intended outcomes which are valued can be realised. For a minute, let us imagine it does not matter what those outcomes might be. What matters is the way in which we approach the task of ensuring there is structure in this messy and confusing world. The rationalist way, we have noted, is to *assume* that there is a workable structure that can be discovered and which will, once put into practice, determine those valued outcomes. Organisation, management and practice then begin to reveal themselves in certain ways. The social constructivist way is to assume nothing except that outcome will be determined through *relationship*. From this world view, organisation, management and practice look quite different. Organisation is not a static, pre-determined and functionalist entity. It is relational, fluid, and negotiated. Management is not rule-bound, technocratic and hierarchical, but guided by procedure, structured through relationship, empowering and democratic. Practice also moves from being rule-bound, imposed, self-serving and oppressive, and instead becomes flexible and responsive, operating within rules which guide rather than determine, is developmental and empowering.

The challenge for policy implementation, however, is the immediacy of policy problems. The need for instant solutions to major predicaments such as budget deficit, means that the rationalist solutions give the appearance of being very attractive. To get it right and so solve a particular problem, is a far more attractive approach than the constructivist response which believes that nothing can be achieved without process, and process takes time - takes for ever, in fact. If policy implementers continue to seek the rationalist way they will continue to encounter implementation deficit. Implementation can only happen through process and that means incrementally. But, adding to the incrementalist message, we must also insist that the process is one of involvement, of participation by all those who have a stake in the process. To deny access to any party, is to disenfranchise them from the participatory process, and marginalise the perspective that would otherwise have contributed to the construction of policy over time, and set up the certainty of resistance on the one hand, or ineffectiveness of outcome on the other. Outcome that is not built upon participation by all stakeholders is unlikely to have meaning for those whose perspective is denied access.

The problem of traditional policy implementation process is that it separates.   There is a demarcation between the makers and the implementers, between implementers in different positions within hierarchical organisations and between implementers and users of services. If social policy is socially constructed, as has been argued, then successful policy implementation will need to maximise opportunities for positive communication between actors involved in the process to ensure effective outcomes. To separate means to fragment the policy process, with the result that different forms of the intended policy will be constructed by different actors in different parts of the hierarchy. The result is that implementation deficit is far more likely to occur.

I have also argued, through Giandomenico Majone (Majone 1989) that learning is an important part of the process of policy implementation. Within both individual and organisational theories of learning the concepts of ownership and meaning are crucial. If knowledge is imposed across hierarchical divides it is likely to be resisted if there is no notion of ownership and meaning. This is another way in which street level bureaucratic behaviour comes into being. Effective policy implementation through management approaches will try and maximise opportunities for individual, group and organisational learning to ensure that knowledge confirmed or created for use in the implementation process has meaning to implementers at all levels, is owned by them, and therefore, has an effect on their practice (Argyris and Schon 1996). Practitioners, we have noted, are able to reframe knowledge that does not have meaning for them so that it fits within their own frame of reference. We have seen how bureaucratic procedures can be rejected as revolting ("they make my gorge rise" - chapter three) or re-framed as a chance for developing an equality of opportunity to resource accessibility, in much the same way that mission statements can be re-framed as supportive of social work values.

If there is no expectation of immediate returns in policy implementation from the process of incrementalism, then nor is there of participation. This too must be a process, moving onwards towards some future of democratic participation. Peter Reason has argued persuasively (Reason 1994a) of the continuing signs that acceptance of this participative world view is gaining ground as a way of making sense of our confusing and fragmented post-modern world.

Future Participation and Care Management

Future participation, as envisaged by Reason (Reason 1994a), provides us with a useful conceptual framework to locate practice in policy implementation, managerial and social work practice, that is likely to be more effective than that described in the empirical work analysed in the early parts of this book. Reason describes future participation as 'a form of consciousness rooted in concrete experience' and 'characterised by self-awareness and self-reflection' (Reason 1994: p.33), so it is a conceptual framework very close to that learning approach for individuals and organisations advocated throughout this book. Quoting Torbert (Torbert 1987), Reason refers to the usefulness of the concept of 're-framing', which describes not just the fact that experience is re-framed but that the individual reflects on the process of framing experience too. In order to engage in such re-framing, an individual needs to adopt both an individual and a collective approach. Re-framing is a methodological concept within social work practice too. To be doing this with colleagues, with management staff, with service users and in the wider community engages care managers in a process of making mutual sense. Re-framing is a form of learning activity for care management that would provide impetus towards future participation.

Another quality of future participation is the active use of imagination (Reason 1994a: p. 35).   Creativity in the process of assessment of human needs has been argued as an important part of effective social work practice that assists practitioners in crossing cultural divides between different perspectives (Brandon and Jordan 1979; England 1984). Imagination, like intuition, is an important force to be released in the creation of effective practice. It is the use of language as a form of classifying and labelling that describes this unitary reality. There is authoritative support from elsewhere (Becker 1963; Lemert 1972; Wood 1985) that this process of labelling 'can be a powerful source of alienation from awareness of participation' (Reason 1994a: p.35). We have already noted the way in which labelling has become a necessary part of care management in the managerial practices of eligibility criteria. These criteria deny opportunities for participation, and service users, in our present case, are, through the imposition of such procedures, constructed as alienated subjects with the construction of the subject being what has been termed a 'false abstraction' (Rojek 1986; p. 69). For care managers and other managers within Social Services Departments, finding imaginative and creative ways of negotiating around these organisational practices is essential if there is to be any chance of meeting one of the principle planks of Community Care policy, which is the involvement of services users, both as individuals in their own assessments, and collectively in service development. Alienated subjects constructed as false abstractions do not possess the authentic humanity to be involved in the construction of anything that will have meaning to vulnerable people.

Reason's final point concerns the nature of humanity as 'self rooted in environment and community' (Reason 1994a: p.37).   The resolution of tension between the individual and the collective, lies at the heart of holistic social work practice for care management as described in Smale et al (Smale et al 1993). In chapter seven we looked at the practice of community profiling, noting the importance and usefulness of seeing the individual as part of their wider community. Participation depends on the continuing development of such practices. To isolate the sense made of someone's existence in an assessment of their needs outside of their being within their wider community means denying a fundamental aspect of who they are. Such individualistic assessments are inauthentic and construct knowledge that will not be useful or useable for developing services that will meet their needs.

There were the beginnings of a developing participation in the co-operative inquiry groups defined in chapter nine. These opportunities need to be extended through the gradual implementation of organisational processes that encourage participation in the form of active critical learning in organisations. Such participation needs to be available and encouraged for all stakeholders in community care policy implementation. In the case of care managers, notably as social workers, in this research, failures of participation will lead to alienation from both the organisational hierarchy and from those people who are reliant upon their services. Effective practice requires participation both through an empowering managerial environment and through the development of empowering social work practices. Given the enormous amounts of human, financial and physical investment that is pooled to construct community care, a failure to nurture participatory practice amounts to a monumental waste of resources. Its continuing disastrous effect on the lives of very vulnerable people means that participation through a mutual learning process is justified on the grounds of economy, efficiency and effectiveness.

Final Words

These deliberations have cast a useful light upon the extent to which policy intentions are inevitably undermined through the unreflective use of discretion by implementers such as care managers in the way that Lipsky describes (Lipsky 1980). Policy implementation needs to be less about developing coercive forms of regulation and more about participation and democratic forms of accountability. It needs to be more about understanding implementation as a co-operative venture in which politicians, managers, professionals, care providers and service users participate in constructing versions of community care within a framework of policy structure. Policy implementation is then best conceptualised as negotiation through participation rather than imposed through hierarchical processes. Versions of community care may not be agreed upon, in the short term, but will at least be debated by actors openly engaged in relationship together. The social construction of knowledge and institutions will happen anyway. The point is whether discretion, which is a key activity, happens in an unbridled and negative way as described by Lipsky and others, and observed in chapter three, or through reflection and as a process of positive developmental learning, as described in chapter nine. Policy implementation, through managerial technique, is then less about imposing scientific rationality on the process of constructing knowledge and meaning and more about facilitating this process in learning organisations. Implementation will be more effective if it is viewed as a participative process of constructing knowledge and working towards agreement on shared aims.

Jaqi Nixon (Nixon 1993) wrote an interesting paper about the policy consensus between senior professionals in the Social Services Inspectorate and Department of Health and senior managers in Social Services Departments. As she notes, senior managers are far more wedded to Community Care changes than their junior colleagues because they were more closely consulted in the development of Community Care and thus feel a degree of ownership of the policy. Everything that we understand about alienation in the workplace would suggest the need for staff lower down in organisations to feel the same sense of ownership when it comes to policy implementation. The illustrative example provided in this book gives us some evidence that this is possible. Social workers can feel a degree of ownership of the policy implementation process if given the kind of opportunities for participation and reflective practice which the co-operative inquiry groups provided. This sort of participation within a learning organisation will transform the use of discretion as a negative, destructive and oppressive activity into positive and developmental practice. Experiments such as that described in chapter nine need to be replicated in other organisations to test out the possibilities both within small parts of organisations as well as in whole agencies.

The implications for my future learning in this area are very much caught up in the concept of learning organisations, even given the wariness around definitions covered in chapter six. My work with care managers in co-operative inquiry groups analysed in chapter nine suggests that if people with a street level bureaucrat role are placed in an environment which to some degree simulates the requirements of a learning organisation, one in which they can actively reflect upon and learn co-operatively from their practice, then they are far more likely to be able to transfer prior knowledge and skills and develop new ways of practising congruent with policy intentions. Secondly, I believe that the co-operative inquiry experiment was a form of inquiry that, if replicated elsewhere, would be likely to enhance learning for practitioners, individually and collectively, in the way the literature suggests that the normative learning organisation would. In this sense co-operative inquiry is a methodology that constructs the learning organisation. Finally, in order to widen the scope of co-operative inquiry and increase the effectiveness of an authority implementing community care, such as a Social Services Department, it would need to be extended to involve service users in the participative inquiry process. This is practice in its infancy, but there is some evidence of beginning success in this (Wiltshire and Swindon User Network 1996; Baldwin 1997; Ramon, S 1998) that needs to be tested out further.

There are still major problems, however, and the most notable is that of ambiguity in policy. Whilst Community Care policy seems to reflect both social work and managerialist discourses, as well as a service user perspective which becomes more influential by the day, there will be something there for social workers, as street level bureaucrats, to resist. Managerialist discursive practice that attempts to override discretion through techniques of scientific management fails to address the opportunities for resistance by actors using their agency, whether as practitioners or service users. If resistance is necessary, in the face of such powerful forms of discourse, then for social workers to engage in a co-operative approach with service users is likely to be far more successful than attempting to resist through the forms of practice we recorded in chapter three. The managerial response may, in the short term, be continued de-professionalisation, and the employment of a workforce trained to apply management-inspired techniques. What would be lost by this in terms of effectiveness of service is another story addressed largely by implication alone in this book. It is an area that opens up possibilities for future participative action research. How alternative forms of training would address the inevitable and continuing use of discretion by non-professional staff remains a central question, although the fundamental tenets of co-operative inquiry - participation, authenticity and creative learning - would seem to point the way. The alternative is that social workers engage collectively (with other stakeholders - managers, service providers AND service users and carers) in a process of constructing practice around policy guidelines. This will allow for a more deliberate and creative process of policy implementation in learning organisations.

Bibliography

Adams, R (1996), *The Personal Social Services*, Addison Wesley Longman, Harlow.

Ahmad, B (1991), *Black Perspective in Social Work*, Venture Press, Birmingham.

Ahmad, W and Atkin, K (1996), *Race and Community Care*, Open University Press, Buckingham.

Ahmed, S (1978), 'Asian Girls and Cultural Conflicts', *Social Work Today*.

Argyris, C and Schon, D (1996), *Organisational Learning II: Theory, Method and Practice*, Addison-Wesley, Reading, Massachusetts.

Audit Commission (1986), *Making a Reality of Community Care*, HMSO, London

Audit Commission (1992a), *The Community Revolution: Personal Social Services and Community Care*, HMSO, London.

Audit Commission (1992b), *The Community Revolution: Managing the Cascade of Change*, HMSO, London.

Bachrach, P and Baratz, M (1970), *Power and Poverty: Theory and Practice*, Oxford University Press, New York.

Baldwin, M (1995), *The Meaning of Care Management*, Social Work Monographs, Norwich.

Baldwin, M (1996a), 'Is Assessment Working? - Policy and Practice in Care Management', *Practice*, Vol. 8 No. 4, pp. 53-59.

Baldwin, M (1996b), 'White Anti-Racism: Is it Really No-Go in Rural Areas?', *Social Work Education*, Vol. 15 No. 1, pp. 18-33.

Baldwin, M (1996c), *The Value of Practice Teaching: Developing the Confidence and Competence of Practice Teachers*, NCH/TCS, Bristol.

Baldwin, M (1997), 'Key Texts in Community Care: The Analysis of Discourse in Government and Government Commissioned Documents which Relate to Care Management', *Social Work and Social Sciences Review*, Vol. 8 No. 2, pp. 76-88.

Bamford, T (1989), 'Discretion and Managerialism' in Shardlow, S (1989), *The Values of Change in Social Work*, Routledge, London.

Bamford, T (1990), *The Future of Social Work*, Macmillan, Basingstoke.

Banks, S (1995), *Ethics and Values in Social Work*, Macmillan, Basingstoke.

Barker, P (1986), *Basic Family Therapy*, 2nd Edition, Collins, London.

Becker, H (1963), *Outsiders: Studies in the Sociology of Deviance*, Free Press, New York.

Beer, S (1985), *Diagnosing the System for Organisations*, John Wiley, Chichester.

Beresford, P and Croft, S (1993), *Citizen Involvement*, Macmillan, Basingstoke.

Beresford, P and Trevillion, S (1995), *Developing Skills in Community Care: A Collaborative Approach*, Arena, Aldershot.

Berger, P and Luckman, T (1966), *The Social Construction of Reality*, Penguin Books, Harmondsworth.

Bookchin, M (1991) *The Ecology of Freedom: the Emergence and Dissolution of Hierarchy*, Black Rose Books; Montreal and New York.

Boud, D Cohen, R and Walker, D (1993), 'Introduction: Understanding Learning from Experience', in Boud, D Cohen, R and Walker, D (eds) (1993), *Using Experience for Learning*, Open University Press, Buckingham

Boud, D Cohen, R and Walker, D (eds) (1993), *Using Experience for Learning*, Open University Press, Buckingham.

Boud, D and Griffiths (eds) (1987), *Appreciating Adults Learning*, Kogan Page, London.

Boud, D Keogh, R and Walker, D (1985), 'Promoting Reflection in Learning: a Model', in Boud et al (1985) *Reflection: Turning Experience into Learning*, Kogan Page, London.

Boud, D Keogh, R and Walker, D (1985), *Reflection: Turning Experience into Learning*, Kogan Page, London.

Boud, D and Walker, D (1993), 'Barriers to Reflection on Experience', in Boud, D Cohen, R and Walker, D (eds) (1993), *Using Experience for Learning*, Open University Press, Buckingham

Boyne, R (1990), *Foucault and Derrida: The Other Side of Reason*, Unwin Hyman, London.

Brandon, D and Jordan, B (1979), *Creative Social Work*, Blackwell, Oxford.

Brandon, D (1979), 'Zen Practice in Social Work' in Brandon, D and Jordan, B (1979), *Creative Social Work*, Blackwell, Oxford.

Braye, S and Preston-Shoot, M (1995), *Empowering Practice in Social Care*, Open University Press, Buckingham.

Brewster, R (1992), 'The New Class? Managerialism and Social Work Education and Training', *Issues in Social Work Education and Training*, Vol.11 No.2, pp 81 - 93.

Brown, A (1992), *Groupwork*, 3rd Edition. Avebury, Aldershot.

Brown, A (1994), 'Groupwork in Britain' in Hanvey, C and Philpot, T, (1994), *Practising Social Work*, Routledge, London.

Burman, E and Parker, I (1993), *Discourse Analytic Research: Repertoire and Readings of Texts in Action*, Routledge, London.

Burrows, R and Loader, B (eds) (1994), *Towards a Post-Fordist Welfare State*, Routledge, London.

Burton, F and Carlen, P (1979), *Official Discourse: on Discourse Analysis, Government Publications, Ideology and the State*, Routledge and Kegan Paul, London.

Carlen (1996) Personal communication.

Carr, W and Kemmis, S (1983), *Becoming Critical: Knowing through Action Research*, Deakin University Press, Victoria.

Carter, P and Jackson, N (1993), 'Modernism, post-modernism and Motivation, or why Expectancy Theory Failed to Come up to Expectation' in Hassard, J and Parker, M (eds) (1993), *Post modernism and Organisations*, Sage, London.

CCETSW (1991), *Rules and Requirements for the Diploma in Social Work*, (CCETSW Paper 30), CCETSW, London.

CCETSW (1991b), *Setting the Context for Change*, CCETSW, London.

CCETSW (1995), *Rules and Requirements for the Diploma in Social Work*, (CCETSW Paper 30: Revised Edition - 'Working Copy'), CCETSW, London.

Challis, D and Davies, B (1986), *Case Management in Community Care: An Evaluated Experiment in the Home Care of the Elderly*, Gower, Aldershot.

Challis (1996), Personal Communication.

Clarke, J (1995), 'Doing the Right Thing? Managerialism and Social Welfare' *Paper for E.S.R.C. 'Professionals in Late Modernity' Seminar*, Imperial College, June 26th 1995.

Clarke, J, Cochrane, A and McLaughlin, E (Eds) (1994), *Managing Social Policy*, Sage, London.

Corrigan, P and Leonard, P (1978), *Social Work Practice under Capitalism: A Marxist Approach*, Macmillan, London.

Curnock, K and Hardiker, P (1979), *Towards Practice Theory: Skills and Methods in Social Assessments*, Routledge and Kegan Paul, London.

Dalrymple, J and Burke, B (1995), *Anti-Oppressive Practice: Social Care and the Law*, Open University Press, Buckingham.

Day, P (1993) Review of Doel and Marsh (1992), in *British Journal of Social Work*,Vol. 23 No. 2, April 1993.

Denzin, N and Lincoln, Y (eds.) (1994), *Handbook of Qualitative Research*, Sage, London.

Department of Health (1989), *Caring for People: Community Care in the Next Decade and Beyond*, HMSO, London.

Department of Health (1990), *Caring for People: Policy Guidance*, HMSO, London.

Department of Health and Social Security (1985), *Social Work Decisions in Child Care: Recent Research Findings and their Implication*, HMSO, London.

De Vries, P (1992), *Unruly Clients: A Study of how Bureaucrats try and fail to transform Gatekeepers, Communists and Preachers into Ideal Beneficiaries*, PhD Thesis, Waneningen Agricultural University, Netherlands.

Dobuzinzkis, L (1992), 'Modernist and Postmodernist Metaphors of the Policy Process: Control and Stability versus Chaos and Reflexive Understanding', *Policy Sciences*, Vol. 5, pp. 355-380.

Doyal, L and Gough, I (1991), *A Theory of Human Need*, Macmillan, Basingstoke.

Doel and Marsh (1992), *Task-Centred Social Work*, Ashgate, Aldershot.

Dominelli, L and Hoogvelt, A (1996), 'Globalization and Technocratization of Social Work', *Critical Social Policy*, Vol. 16 No. 2, pp. 45-62.

Eliassen, K and Kooiman, J (1993), *Managing Public Organisations: Lessons from Contemporary European Experience*, Sage, London.

Ellis, K (1993), *Squaring the Circle: User and Carer Participation in Needs Assessment*, Joseph Rowntree, York.

England, H (1986), *Social Work as Art*, Allen and Unwin, London.

Epstein, L (1980), *Helping People: The Task-Centred Approach*, CV Mosby, St Louis.

Evans, C (1997), *'From Bobble Hats to Red Jackets': A History of the first 5 years of Wiltshire and Swindon Users' Network*, WCCUIN, Devizes.

Everitt, A and Hardiker, P (1996), *Evaluating for Good Practice*, Macmillan, Basingstoke.

Everitt, A Hardiker, P Littlewood, J and Mullender, A (1992), *Applied Research for Better Practice*, Macmillan, Basingstoke.

Farnham, D and Horton, S (1993), *Managing the New Public Services*, Macmillan, Basingstoke.

Fischer, F (1993), 'Reconstructing Policy Analysis: A Post-Positivist Perspective', *Policy Sciences*, Vol. 25, pp. 333-339.

Fisher, M (1997),'Research, Knowledge and Practice in Community Care', *Issues in Social Work Education*, Vol. 17 No. 2,pp. 17-30.

Flynn, N (1990), *Public Sector Management*, Harvester Wheatsheaf, Hemel Hempstead.

Foddy, W (1993), *Constructing Questions for Interviews and Questionnaires: Theory and Practice in Social Research*, Cambridge University Press, Cambridge.

Fook, J (1996), 'Making Connections: Reflective Practices and Formal Theories', in Fook, J (ed.) (1996), *The Reflective Researcher: Social Workers' Theories of Practice Research*, Allen and Unwin, St. Leonard's, Australia.

Fook, J (ed.) (1996), *The Reflective Researcher: Social Workers' Theories of Practice Research*, Allen and Unwin, St. Leonard's, Australia.

Foucault (1977), *Language, Counter-Memory, Practice*, Blackwell, quoted in Macdonnell (1986), *Theories of Discourse*, Blackwell, Oxford.

Freire, P (1972), *Pedagogy of the Oppressed*, Penguin, London.

Gerding, G (1993), 'Public Managers in the Middle', in Eliassen, K and Kooiman, J (1993), *Managing Public Organisations: Lessons from Contemporary European Experience*, Sage, London.

Giddens, A (1976), *New Rules of Sociological Method*, Hutchinson, London.

Gilroy, P (1987), *There ain't no Black in the Union Jack*, Hutchinson, London.

Goffman (1961), *Asylums: Essays on the Social Situation of Mental Patients and Other Inmates*, Pelican Books, Harmondsworth.

Goldberg, E. Matilda Gibbons, J and Sinclair, I (1984), *Problems, Tasks and Outcomes*, Allen and Unwin, London.

Goodsell, C (ed.) (1981), *The Public Encounter: Where State and Citizen Meet*, Indiana University Press, Bloomington.

Gould, N (1992), 'Anti-Racist Social Work; A Framework for Teaching and Action', *Issues in Social Work Education*, Vol. 11.

Gould, N and Taylor, I (1996), *Reflective Learning for Social Work*, Arena, Aldershot.

Green, R and Zinke, R (1993), 'The Rhetorical Way of Knowing and Public Administration', *Administration and Society, Vol. 25 No. 3, pp. 317-334.*

Gregg, R (1994), 'Explorations of Pregnancy and Choice in a High-Tech Age', in Riessman, C (ed.) (1994), *Qualitative Studies in Social Work Research*, Sage, London.

Griffiths, Sir R (1988), *Community Care: Agenda for Action*, (The Griffiths Report), HMSO, London.

Guba, E (ed.) (1990), *The Paradigm Dialog*, Sage, London.

Hall, A (1974), *The Point of Entry*, Allen and Unwin, London.

Ham, C and Hill, M (1993), *The Policy Process in the Modern Capitalist State*, 2nd Edition, Harvester Wheatsheaf, Hemel Hempstead.

Hamilton, G (1951), *Theory and Practice of Social Casework*, 2nd Edition, Columbia University Press, New York.

Hammersley, M and Atkinson, P (1995), *Ethnography*, 2nd Edition, Routledge, London.

Hanvey, C and Philpot, T, (1994), Practising Social Work. Routledge, London.

Hardiker, P and Barker, M (1979), *Theories of Practice in Social Work*, Academic Press, London.

Harding, T and Beresford, P (1996), *The Standards We Expect: What Service Users and Carers Want from Social Services Workers*, National Institute for Social Work, London.

Harre, R (1981),'The Positivist-Empiricist Approach and its Alternatives' in Reason, P and Rowan, J (1981a), *Human Inquiry: A Sourcebook of New Paradigm Research*, John Wiley, Chichester.

Harrison, S and Pollitt, C (1994), *Controlling Health Professionals: The Future of Work and Organization*, Blackwell, Oxford.

Hasenfeld, Y and Steinmetz, D (1981), 'Client-Official Encounters in Social Services Agencies' in Goodsell, C (ed.) (1981), *The Public Encounter: Where State and Citizen Meet*, Indiana University Press, Bloomington.

Hassard, J and Parker, M (eds) (1993), *Post modernism and Organisations*, Sage, London.

Hawtin, M (1994), *Community Profiling: Auditing Social Needs*, Open University Press, Buckingham.

Henwood, M (1992), *Through a Glass Darkly: Community Care and Elderly People*, King's Fund Institute, London.

Heron, J (1981), 'Philosophical basis for a new paradigm', in Reason, P and Rowan, J (1981a), *Human Inquiry: A Sourcebook of New Paradigm Research*, John Wiley, Chichester.

Heron, J (1996), *Co-operative Inquiry, Research into the Human Condition*, Sage, London.

Heron, J and Reason, P (1997), 'A Participatory Inquiry Paradigm' in *Qualitative Inquiry*, September 1997.

Heron J and Reason, P (1997), 'A Participatory Inquiry Paradigm', *Qualitative Inquiry*, 1997.

Hill, M (ed.) (1993a), *New Agendas in the Study of the Policy Process*, Harvester Wheatsheaf, Hemel Hempstead.

Hill, M (ed.) (1993b), *The Policy Process: A Reader*, Harvester Wheatsheaf, Hemel Hempstead.

Hill, M (1993c), *Understanding Social Policy*, 4th Edition, Blackwell, Oxford.

Hill, M (ed.) (1997a), *The Policy Process: A Reader*,2nd Edition, Prentice Hall, London.

Hill, M (1997b), *The Policy Process in the Modern State*, 3rd Edition, Prentice Hall, Hemel Hempstead.

Hill, M and Bramley, G (1986), *Analysing Social Policy*, Blackwell, Oxford.

HMSO (1990), *National Health Service and Community Care Act*, HMSO, London.

Hogwood, B and Gunn, L (1984), *Policy Analysis for the Real World*, Oxford University Press, London.

Hollis, F (1972), *Casework: A Psycho-social Therapy*, 2nd Edition, Random House, New York.

Howe, D (1987), *An Introduction to Social Work Theory*, Wildwood House, Aldershot.

Howe, D (1989), *Consumers' View of Family Therapy*, Gower, Aldershot.

Howe, D (1994), 'Modernity, Postmodernity and Social Work', *British Journal of Social Work*, Vol. 24, pp. 513-532.

Howe, D (1996), "Surface and depth in social work practice" in Parton, N (1996).

Hudson, B and Macdonald, G (1986), *Behavioural Social Work: an Introduction*, Macmillan, London.

Hudson, B (1989), 'Michael Lipsky and Street Level Bureaucracy: A Neglected Perspective', in Hill, M (ed.) (1997a), *The Policy Process: A Reader*, 2nd Edition, Prentice Hall, London.

Hughes, B (1995), *Older People and Community Care: Critical Theory and Practice*, Open University Press, Buckingham.

Hugman, R (1991), *Power in Caring Professions*, Macmillan, Basingstoke.

Hugman, R and Smith, D (eds) (1995), *Ethical Issues in Social Work*, R outledge, London.

Jackson, M (1991), *Systems Methodology for the Management Sciences*, Plenum, London.

James, A (1994), *Managing to Care: Public Service and the Market*, Longman, Harlow.

Jordan, B (1979), *Helping in Social Work*, Routledge and Kegan Paul, London.

Jordan, B (1984), *Invitation to Social Work*, Blackwell, Oxford.

Jordan, B (1990), *Social Work in an Unjust Society*, Harvester Wheatsheaf, Hemel Hempstead.

Kemmis, S and McTaggart (1982), *The Action Research Planner*, Deakin University Press, Victoria.

Kolb, D (1984), *Experiential Learning: Experience as the Source of Learning and Development*, Prentice-Hall, Englewood Cliffs, New Jersey.

Krill, D (1978), *Existential Social Work*, Free Press, New York.

Laragy, C (1996), 'Finding a methodology to meet the needs of research: moving towards a participatory approach' in Fook, J (ed.) (1996), *The Reflective Researcher: Social Workers' Theories of Practice Research*, Allen and Unwin, St. Leonard's, Australia.

Le Grand, J and Bartlett, W (eds) (1993), *Quasi Markets and Social Policy*, Macmillan, Basingstoke.

Lemert, E (1972), *Human Deviance, Social Problems and Social Control*, 2nd Edition, Prentice-Hall, New Jersey.

Lewis, J and Glennerster, H (1996), *Implementing the New Community Care*, Open University, Buckingham.

Lindblom, C (1988), *Democracy and Market Systems*, Norwegian University Press, Oslo.

Lindblom, C and Woodhouse, EJ (1993), *The Policy Making Process*, Prentice Hall, Englewood Cliffs, New Jersey.

Lindlof, T (1995), *Qualitative Communication Research Methods*, Sage, London.

Lipsky (1980), *Street Level Bureaucrats: Dilemmas of the Individual in Public Services*, Russell Sage Foundation, New York.

Long, N and Long, A (eds)(1992), *Battlefields of Knowledge: The Interlocking of Theory and Practice in Social Research and Development*, Routledge, London.

Lukes, S (1974), *Power: A Radical View*, Macmillan, Basingstoke.

Lyotard, J-F (1986), *The Postmodern Condition: A Report on Knowledge*, (Translation by Bennington, G and Massumi, B), Manchester University Press, Manchester.

Macdonnell (1986), *Theories of Discourse*, Blackwell, Oxford.

Majone, G (1989), *Evidence, Argument and Persuasion in the Policy Process*, Yale University Press, New Haven.

Malin, N (ed) (1994), *Implementing Community Care*, Open University, Buckingham.

McGill, I and Beaty, L (1995), *Action Learning: A guide for professional, management and educational development*, 2nd Edition, Kogan Page, London.

McKevitt, D and Lawton, A (eds) (1994), *Public Sector Management: Theory, Critique and Practice*, Sage, London.

McNiff, J with Whitehead, J Laidlaw, M (1992), *Creating a Good Social Order through Action Research*, Hyde Publications, Poole.

Means, R and Smith, R (1994), *Community Care: Policy and Practice*, Macmillan, Basingstoke.

Middleton, L (1997), *The Art of Assessment*, Venture Press, Birmingham.

Mintzberg, H (1989), *Mintzberg on Management: Inside our Strange World of Organizations.*, Free Press, New York.

Mladenka, K (1981), 'Responsive Performance by Public Officials' in Goodsell, C (ed.) (1981), *The Public Encounter: Where State and Citizen Meet*, Indiana University Press, Bloomington.

Morgan, C and Murgatroyd, S (1994), *Total Quality Management in the Public Sector*, Open University Press, Buckingham.

Morrice, J (1976), *Crisis Intervention: Studies in Community Care*, Pergamon, London.

Morris, J (1991), *Pride Against Prejudice: Transforming Attitudes to Disability*, The Women's Press, London.

Morris, J (1993), *Community Care or Independent Living?*, Joseph Rowntree, York.

Morris, J (1995), *The Shape of Things to Come? user-led social services*, Social Services Forum, Paper No.3, London National Institute for Social Work .

Nixon, J (1993), 'Implementation in the hands of Senior Managers: Community Care in Britain', in Hill, M (ed.) (1993a), *New Agendas in the Study of the Policy Process*, Harvester Wheatsheaf, Hemel Hempstead.

O'Hagan, K (1986), *Crisis Intervention in Social Services*, Macmillan, London.

Oliver, M (1996), *Understanding Disability: From Theory to Practice*, Macmillan, Basingstoke.

Parad, H (ed.) (1965), *Crisis Intervention: Selected Reading*, Family Services Association of America, New York.

Parker, I (1989), 'Discourse and Power', in Shotter, J and Gergen K (eds) (1989), *Tests of Identity*, Sage, London.

Parker, I (1992), *Discourse Dynamics: Critical Analysis for Social and Individual Psychology*, Routledge, London.

Parton, N (1994), 'Problems of Government, (Post) Modernity and Social Work', *British Journal of Social Work*, Vol. 24, pp. 9-32.

Parton, N (ed.) (1996), *Social Theory, Social Change and Social Work*, Routledge, London.

Payne, M (1991), *Modern Social Work Theory: A Critical Introduction*, Macmillan, Basingstoke.

Payne, M (1993), *Linkages: Effective Networking in Social Care*, Whiting and Birch, London.

Payne, M (1995), *Social Work and Community Care*, Macmillan, Basingstoke.

Peters, B. Guy (1993), 'Managing the Hollow State' in Eliassen, K and Kooiman, J (1993), *Managing Public Organisations: Lessons from Contemporary European Experience*, Sage, London.

Pollitt, C (1990), *Managerialism and the Public Services: The Anglo-American Experience*, Blackwell, Oxford.

Pollitt, C (1993), *Managerialism and the Public Services*, 2nd Edition, Blackwell, Oxford.

Pottage, D and Evans, M (1994), *The Competent Workplace: The View from Within*, NISW, London.

Potter, J (1988), 'Consumerism and the Public Sector: How Well does the Coat Fit?' in McKevitt, D and Lawton, A (1994), *Public Sector Management: Theory, Critique and Practice*, Sage, London.

Potter, J (1996), *Representing Reality: Discourse, Rhetoric and Social Construction*, Sage, London.

Power, M (1994), *The Audit Explosion*, Demos, London.

Pressman, J and Wildavsky, A (1973), *Implementation*, University of California Press, Berkeley, California.

Preston-Shoot, M (1987), *Effective Groupwork*, Macmillan, London.

Ramcharan, P Roberts, G Grant, G and Borland, J (eds) (1997), *Empowerment in Everyday Life*, Jessica Kingsley, London.

Ramon, S (1998), Personal Communication.

Ransom, S and Stewart, J (1994), *Management for the Public Domain: Enabling the Learning Society*, Macmillan, Basingstoke .

Reason, P (ed.) (1988), *Human Inquiry in Action: Developments in New Paradigm Research*, Sage, London.

Reason, P (ed.) (1994a), *Participation in Human Inquiry*, Sage, London.

Reason, P (1994b), 'Three Approaches to Participative Inquiry' in Denzin, N and Lincoln, Y (eds.) (1994), *Handbook of Qualitative Research*, Sage, London.

Reason, P (1996), 'Reflections on the Purposes of Human Inquiry' *Qualitative Inquiry*, Vol. 2 No. 1, pp. 15-28.

Reason, P and Heron, J (1995), 'Co-operative Inquiry', in Smith, J Harre, R and Langenhove, L (1995), *Rethinking Methods in Psychology*, Sage, London.

Reason, P and Marshall, J (1987), 'Research as a Personal Process' in Boud, D and Griffiths (eds) (1987), *Appreciating Adults Learning*, Kogan Page, London.

Reason, P and Rowan, J (1981a), *Human Inquiry: A Sourcebook of New Paradigm Research*, John Wiley, Chichester.

Reason, P and Rowan, J (1981b), 'Issues of validity in new paradigm research' in Reason, P and Rowan, J (1981a), *Human Inquiry: A Sourcebook of New Paradigm Research*, John Wiley, Chichester.

Reid, W and Epstein, L (1972), *Task Centred Casework*, Columbia University Press, New York.

Riessman, C (ed.) (1994), *Qualitative Studies in Social Work Research*, Sage, London.

Rogers, C (1951), *Client-Centred Therapy: Its Current Practice, Implications and Theory*, Constable, London.

Rojek, C (1986), 'The 'Subject' in Social Work', *British Journal of Social Work*, *Vol. 16, pp. 65-77*.

Rojek, C, Peacock, G and Collins, S (1988),   *Social Work and Received Ideas*, Routledge, London.

Sadd, J (1995), Wiltshire and Swindon Service User Network, Personal Communication.

Satyamurti, C (1981), *Occupational Survival: The Case of the Local Authority Social Worker*, Blackwell, Oxford.

Schon, D (1984), *The Reflective Practitioner: How Professionals Think in Action*, Basic Books, New York.

Schon, D (1987), *Educating the Reflective Practitioner*, Jossey-Bass, San Francisco.

Schram, S (1993), 'Postmodern Policy Analysis: Discourse and Identity in Welfare Policy', *Policy Sciences*, Vol. 26, pp. 249-270.

Schurandt, T (1990), 'Paths to Inquiry in the Social Disciplines: Scientific, Constructivist and Critical Theory Methodologies' in Guba, E (ed) (1990), *The Paradigm Dialog*, Sage, London.

Senge, P (1990), *The Fifth Discipline: The Art and Practice of the Learning Organisation*, Random House, London.

Shardlow, S (1989), *The Values of Change in Social Work*, Routledge, London.

Shaw, I (1996), *Evaluating in Practice*, Arena, Aldershot.

Sheldon, B (1986), 'Social Work Effectiveness Experiments: Review and Implications', *British Journal of Social Work*, Vol. 16 No. 2, pp.223-242.

Shepperd, M (1995), *Care Management and the New Social Work: a Critical Analysis*, Whiting and Birch, London.

Shotter, J and Gergen K (eds) (1989), *Tests of Identity*, Sage, London.

Silverman, D (1993), *Interpreting Qualitative Data: Methods for Analyzing Talk, Text and Interaction*, Sage, London.

Smale, G Tuson, G with Biehal, N and Marsh, P (1993), *Empowerment, Assessment, Care Management and the Skilled Worker*, HMSO, London.

Smith, D (1987), 'The Limits of Positivism in Social Work Research', *British Journal of Social Work, Vol. 17, pp. 401-416*.

Smith, G and May, D (1980), 'The Artificial Debate between Rational and Incrementalist Models of Decision Making' in Hill, M (ed.) (1993a), *New Agendas in the Study of the Policy Process*, Harvester Wheatsheaf, Hemel Hempstead.

Smith, J Harre, R and Langenhove, L (1995), *Rethinking Methods in Psychology*, Sage, London.

Social Services Committee (1985), *Second Report: Community Care*, House of Commons Paper 13-1, HMSO, London.

Social Services Inspectorate/Social Work Services Group (1991a),   *Care Management and Assessment: Managers' Guide*, HMSO, London.

Social Services Inspectorate/Social Work Services Group (1991b), *Care Management and Assessment: Practitioners' Guide*, HMSO, London.

Souza, A (with Ramcharan, P) (1997), 'Everything You Ever Wanted to Know About Down's Syndrome, but Never Bothered to Ask', in Ramcharan, P Roberts, G Grant, G and Borland, J (eds) (1997), *Empowerment in Everyday Life*, Jessica Kingsley, London.

Soyland, AJ (1994), *Psychology as Metaphor*, Sage, London.

Steir, F (1991), *Research and Reflexivity*, Sage, London.

Stenson, K (1993), 'Social Work Discourse and the Social Work Interview', *Economy and Society, Vol. 22 No. 1, pp 42-76.*

Stevenson, O and Parsloe, P (1993), *Community Care and Empowerment*, Joseph Rowntree, York.

Stewart, J and Ransom, S (1988), 'Management in the Public Domain' in McKevitt, D and Lawton, A (eds) (1994), *Public Sector Management: Theory, Critique and Practice*, Sage, London.

Stone, C (1981), 'Attitudinal tendencies among officials' in Goodsell, C (ed.) (1981), *The Public Encounter: Where State and Citizen Meet*, Indiana University Press, Bloomington.

Street, E and Dryden, W (1988), *Family Therapy in Britain*, Open University Press, Buckingham.

Taylor, M Hoyes, L Lart, R and Means, R (1992), *User Empowerment in Community Care: Unravelling the Issues*, School for Advanced Urban Studies, Bristol.

Thompson, N (1991), *Crisis Intervention Re-visited*, Pepar, Birmingham.

Thompson, N (1995), *Theory and Practice in Health and Social Welfare*, Open University, Buckingham.

Torbert, W (1987), *Managing the Corporate Dream; Restructuring for Long-term Success*, Jones-Irwin, Homewood, IL.

Trevillion, S (1992), *Caring in the Community: A Networking Approach to Community Partnership*, Longman, Harlow.

Tsang, E (1997), 'Organisational learning and the Learning organisation: A Dichotomy between Descriptive and Prescriptive Research' , *Human Relations*, Vol. 50 No. 1, pp. 73-89.

Wagner (1988), *Residential Care: A Positive Choice*, HMSO, London.

Walsh, K (1995), *Public Services and Market Mechanisms: Competition, Contracting and the New Public Management*, Macmillan, Basingstoke.

Warde, A 'Consumers, Consumption and Post-Fordism', in Burrows, R and Loader, B (eds) (1994), *Towards a Post-Fordist Welfare State*, Routledge, London.

Watters, C (1996), 'Representation and Realities: Black People, Community Care and Mental Illness', in Ahmad, W and Atkin, K (1996), *'Race' and Community Care*, Open University Press, Buckingham.

Whittington, C and Holland, R (1985), 'A Framework for Theory in Social Work', *Issues in Social Work Education*, Vol 5. No. 1, pp. 25-50.

Williams, F (1994), 'Social Relations, Welfare and post-Fordism', in Burrows, R and Loader, B (eds) (1994), *Towards a Post-Fordist Welfare State*, Routledge, London.

Wilmot, S (1997), *The Ethics of Community Care*, Cassell, London.

Wiltshire and Swindon Users' Network (1996), *'I am in control': Research into Users' Views of the Wiltshire Independent Living Fund*, WCCUIN, Devizes.
Wood, G (ed.) (1985), *Labelling in Development Policy: Essays in Honour of Bernard Schaffer*, Sage, London.